Small's Practical Guide to

Botulinum
Toxin
Procedures

SECOND EDITION

Small's Practical Guide to

Botulinum Toxin Procedures

SECOND EDITION

Series Editor

Rebecca Small MD, FAAFP
Associate Clinical Professor,
Family and Community Medicine,
University of California,
San Francisco, California

Director, Medical Aesthetics Training,
Natividad Medical Center,
Family Medicine Residency Program–UCSF Affiliate,
Salinas, California

Medical Director,
RSMD Medical Aesthetics,
Private Practice,
Capitola, California

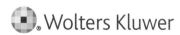
 Wolters Kluwer

Philadelphia · Baltimore · New York · London
Buenos Aires · Hong Kong · Sydney · Tokyo

Acquisitions Editor: Joe Cho
Senior Development Editor: Ashley Fischer
Editorial Coordinator: Sunmerrilika Baskar
Marketing Manager: Kirsten Watrud
Production Project Manager: Bridgett Dougherty
Design Coordinator: Stephen Druding
Manufacturing Coordinator: Lisa Bowling
Prepress Vendor: Straive

Second Edition

Cataloging-in-Publication Data available on request from the Publisher

ISBN: 978-1-9751-9285-3

This material is a compilation of the author's clinical experiences intended exclusively for qualified licensed healthcare providers trained in medical aesthetic treatments. While efforts have been made to ensure the accuracy of this information, it is provided "as is." Readers are solely responsible for consulting a qualified health care professional and independently verifying all information and data before treating patients or employing any therapies described in this publication. This work is solely for informational and educational purposes and does not constitute medical advice or guidance and should not be interpreted as such by readers.

The author, editor, and publisher disclaim any and all warranties, express or implied, including those related to the adequacy, reliability, accuracy, completeness, or currency of the content of this work and associated media. Treating healthcare professionals, not the author, editor, or publisher, are solely responsible for the use of this work, including medical judgment and resulting diagnoses, treatments, and outcomes. This work does not replace individual patient assessments conducted by healthcare professionals, considering all relevant factors. It is the professional responsibility of the medical provider to determine the appropriate application of the presented information in a particular situation, and to comply with relevant laws and regulations governing the drugs, devices, and treatments they offer.

Given continuous, rapid advances in medical science and health information, independent professional verification of medical diagnoses, indications, appropriate pharmaceutical selections and dosages, and treatment options should be made and healthcare professionals should consult a variety of sources.

Off-label uses of FDA-approved products are described. When prescribing medication, health care providers should consult the manufacturer's package insert, verifying, among other things, conditions of use, indications, warnings, precautions, side effects, and identify any changes in indications, dosage, contraindications and any added warnings and precautions. This is especially important for new, infrequently used, or narrowly therapeutic range medications. It is the responsibility of the reader to ascertain the FDA status of each drug or device planned for use in their clinical practice.

To the maximum extent permitted by applicable law, readers assume all risks and liabilities associated with the use of this information, and the author, editor, and publisher assume no responsibility for any injury or damage to persons or property, whether under product liability, negligence law or otherwise, arising from any reference to or use of this work or associated media.

shop.lww.com

About the Author

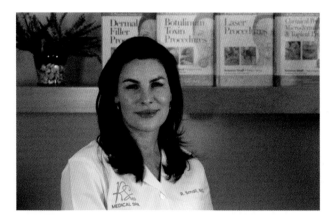

Rebecca Small, MD, is a leading authority in combining nonsurgical medical aesthetic therapies to slow the signs of aging. She is a graduate of Cambridge University, England, and Harvard Medical School. Dr. Small is an Associate Clinical Professor at the University of California, San Francisco (UCSF), School of Medicine, where she trains Plastic Surgery and Family Medicine residents. She codeveloped and precepts the Nonsurgical Medical Aesthetics curriculum for the Plastic and Reconstructive Surgery Core Surgical Curriculum (PRSCSC) at UCSF School of Medicine. She is also the Director of Medical Aesthetics Training for Dominican Hospital in Santa Cruz and Natividad Medical Center in Salinas, California.

Dr. Small's *Practical Guide* textbook series covering botulinum toxins, dermal fillers, lasers, and medical skincare has been translated into 6 languages and has sold more than 20,000 copies worldwide. These textbooks consistently achieve "#1 Best Seller" in Amazon's Plastic Surgery, Dermatology, and Laser Medicine categories, garnering more than 700 5-star reviews.

For more than 10 years, Dr. Small has trained residents in her office as part of their core aesthetic medicine and dermatology rotation, and her elective rotations are consistently oversubscribed. Dr. Small's unique ability to adapt her didactic instruction, demonstration, and hands-on precepting to the student has earned her outstanding evaluation ratings from UCSF Family Medicine and Plastic Surgery residents and Nurse Practitioners.

Dr. Small has volunteered at her local hospital in the Tattoo Removal Program for over a decade, removing visible tattoos that are a barrier to employment. In addition to teaching and writing, Dr. Small is the Medical Director at her private practice, RSMD Medical Aesthetics, in Santa Cruz, California, where she has been providing nonsurgical medical aesthetic patient care for over 15 years.

Foreword

As the Associate Program Director of the University of California, San Francisco (UCSF), Plastic Surgery Residency program, I am responsible for developing the residents' curriculum and ensuring they obtain the knowledge and procedural excellence expected of a plastic surgeon. It has been our good fortune to have Rebecca Small, MD, participate in the development and implementation of our formal outpatient aesthetic program, now part of the UCSF Plastic Surgery Resident's Core Curriculum. I have worked side-by-side with her in our UCSF Skills Labs and have observed Dr. Small's lectures, demonstrations, and precepting of injectable procedures. In the 10 years that I have been on the faculty at UCSF, I've observed many instructors and training programs and I can unreservedly say that Dr. Small is the best instructor of botulinum toxin and dermal filler outpatient procedures I've seen.

Her lectures are rigorous and evidence-based and combine information from current literature together with pearls from her years in clinical practice. She builds students' confidence by identifying Safety Zones for treatment and thoroughly discussing complications and strategies for their management. Residents quickly pick up techniques observing Dr. Small's demonstrations as she focuses on relevant anatomy, provides technique pearls, and answers questions—all while maintaining a patient-centered approach to ensure the best possible procedural experience for the patient.

Like her training, these books are evidence and experience based. They are refreshingly to the point and accurate, and the information presented is easy and quick to assimilate, which prepares the learner to take the next step of performing hands-on procedures. Tips from years in clinical practice shorten the learning curve for new injectors and can help refine injection techniques for the most experienced. The use of case-based learning, which is the gold standard for health care provider education, is a welcome addition to this book, allowing providers to apply and adapt techniques to patients with varied anatomy.

In short, Dr. Small is an expert educator and aesthetic clinician. We have invited her to participate in the UCSF Plastic Surgery Core Curriculum to train our residents because she has the depth of knowledge, teaching ability, clinical experience, and procedural skill to train outpatient aesthetic procedures to plastic surgeons. I highly recommend her books in preparation for any aesthetic procedure training and as a resource for providers already performing aesthetic injections seeking to improve their skills.

Esther A. Kim, MD, FACS
Associate Professor, Division of Plastic and Reconstructive Surgery
Director, UCSF Gender Affirming Surgery
Associate Program Director, UCSF Plastic Surgery Residency
Codirector, UCSF Microsurgery Fellowship
University of California
San Francisco, California

As a lecturer, editor, author, and medical reviewer, I have had ample opportunity to evaluate many speakers as well as extensive medical literature. After reviewing this series of books on cosmetic procedures by Rebecca Small, MD, I have concluded that it has to be one of the best and most detailed, yet practical, presentation of the topics that I have ever encountered. As a physician whose practice is limited solely to providing office procedures, I see great value in these texts for clinicians and the patients they serve.

The goal of medical care is to make patients feel better and to help them experience an improved quality of life that extends for an optimal, productive period. Interventions may be directed at the emotional/psychiatric, medical/physical, or self-image areas.

For many physicians, performing medical procedures provides excitement in the practice of medicine. The ability to see what has been accomplished in a concrete way provides the positive feedback we all seek in providing care. Sometimes, it involves removing a tumor. At other times, it may be performing a screening procedure to be sure no disease is present. Maybe it is making patients feel better about their appearance. For whatever reason, the "hands on" practice of medicine is more rewarding for some practitioners.

In the late 1980s and early 1990s, there was resurgence in the interest of performing procedures in primary care. It did not involve hospital procedures but rather those that could be performed in the office. Coincidentally, patients also became interested in less invasive procedures such as laparoscopic cholecystectomy, endometrial ablation, and more. The desire for plastic surgery "extreme makeovers" waned, as technology was developed to provide a gentle, more kind approach to "rejuvenation."

Baby boomers were increasing in numbers and wanted to maintain their youthful appearance. This not only improved self-image but it also helped when competing with a younger generation both socially and in the workplace.

These forces then of technological advances, provider interest, and patient desires have led to a huge increase in and demand for "minimally invasive procedures" that has extended to all of medicine. Plastic surgery and aesthetic procedures have indeed been affected by this movement. There have been many new procedures developed in just the last 10–15 years along with constant updates and improvements. As patient demand has soared for these new treatments, physicians have found that there is a whole new world of procedures they need to incorporate into their practice if they are going to provide the latest in aesthetic services.

Rebecca Small, MD, the editor and author of this series of books on cosmetic procedures, has been at the forefront of the aesthetic procedures movement. She has written extensively and conducted numerous workshops to help others learn the latest techniques. She has the practical experience to know just what the physician needs to develop a practice and provides "the latest and the best" in these books. Using her knowledge of the field, she has selected the topics wisely to include:

- *A Practical Guide to: Botulinum Toxin Procedures*
- *A Practical Guide to: Dermal Filler Procedures*
- *A Practical Guide to: Skin Care Procedures and Products*
- *A Practical Guide to: Cosmetic Laser Procedures*

Dr. Small does not just provide a cursory, quick review of these subjects. Rather, they are an in-depth practical guide to performing these procedures. The emphasis here should be on "practical" and "in depth." There is no extra esoteric waste of words, yet every procedure is explained in a clear, concise, useful format that allows practitioners of all levels of experience to learn and gain from reading these texts.

The basic outline of these books consists of the pertinent anatomy, the specific indications and contraindications, specific how to diagram and explanations on performing the procedures, complications and how to deal with them, tables with comparisons and amounts of materials needed, before and after patient instructions as well as consent forms (an immense time-saving feature), sample procedure notes, and a list of supply sources. An extensive updated bibliography is provided in each text for further reading. Photos are abundant depicting the performance of the procedures as well as before and after results. These comprehensive texts are clearly written for the practitioner who wants to "learn everything" about the topics covered. Patients definitely desire these procedures, and Dr. Small has provided the information to meet the physician demand to learn them.

For those interested in aesthetic procedures, these books will be a godsend. Even for those not so interested in performing the procedures described, the reading is easy and interesting and will update the reader on what is currently available so they might better advise their patients.

Dr. Small has truly written a one-of-a-kind series of books on Cosmetic Procedures. It is my prediction that it will be received very well and be most appreciated by all who make use of it.

John L. Pfenninger, MD, FAAFP
Founder and President, The Medical Procedures Center
PC Founder and Senior Consultant, The National Procedures Institute
Clinical Professor of Family Medicine, Michigan State College of Human Medicine

Preface

Over the years, I've trained clinicians from many different specialties with a wide range of skill and knowledge levels. From these experiences, I have developed a method of training using this book as the foundation for didactic instruction, demonstration, and hands-on injection that is successful for both beginners and experienced clinicians. My goal is to help clinicians shorten their learning curve, gain procedural expertise safely, and advance from training to practice with confidence, regardless of previous medical aesthetics experience.

The first edition of this book has been an excellent resource for plastic surgeons, dermatologists, primary care providers, nurse practitioners, physician associates/assistants, and residents interested in performing outpatient aesthetic procedures. Since its original publication, there has been a surge in patient demand for nonsurgical medical aesthetic procedures that has created a tremendous opportunity for clinicians who want to provide aesthetic care. The trend in medicine has shifted away from one-time surgical interventions toward minimally invasive procedures that offer more subtle enhancements and require less recovery time. According to the American Society for Aesthetic Plastic Surgery, over 4.5 million injectable procedures are performed in the United States annually, and the total number of injectable procedures performed globally is projected to grow by up to 14% per year (McKinsey, USA). Botulinum toxin procedures have been, and remain, the most common aesthetic procedure requested by adults of all ages and genders.

This book is the first in my series on nonsurgical medical aesthetic procedures. To ensure this second edition remained a truly practical guide, I utilized feedback from faculty, residents, advanced practice clinicians, and colleagues, together with observations from teaching and my own experience with patients as my practice has evolved over time. Additions and improvements were made to help providers refine and customize botulinum toxin treatments to best meet the needs of their patients.

At the beginning of each chapter, I present Key Points so readers can quickly identify which treatment areas can be performed by novice injectors and which require more skill and are appropriate for experienced injectors. I have added new chapters on advanced areas that are often not covered in other textbooks, such as masseter, Nefertiti lift, necklace lines, chest lines, and nasal tip elevation. A chapter on treatment of facial asymmetry is included that provides a straightforward approach for assessing and managing hyper- and hypodynamic asymmetries. A new approach for using high-dose toxins that extend the duration of botulinum toxin effects has been added as well.

Detailed illustrations of anatomy are enhanced by layering diagrams of facial musculature on top of real patient photos to accurately identify the muscles for injection utilizing surface anatomic landmarks. To reduce the risk of complications, I have added new illustrations highlighting targeted muscles and labelled photos that demonstrate optimal placement and Safety Zones for injections in each chapter. Injection depths for each treatment site have also been added to further guide the reader. A Quick Guide to Dosing with the starting doses for all facial areas has been added at the front of the book for easy reference, and a summary table of complementary treatments that can be combined with botulinum toxin to enhance results is also included.

Patient assessment and follow-up sections are more comprehensive. They include discussion of adjacent muscles to help avoid complications, and review treatment of multiple muscles to help balance opposing muscle functions and create facial harmony. This edition emphasizes approaches that can be used to achieve a natural pattern of aging without the appearance of overtreatment. Moreover, the benefit of working on facial features based on patient preference rather than adhering to conventions of "masculine" and "feminine" beauty are also discussed. I have included over 20 cases from patients in my practice with diverse anatomy and a variety of genders and ethnicities, to help clinicians apply techniques learned from this book to their practice.

The knowledge and guidance presented in this book provides new and experienced injectors with a solid foundation and best practices for performing botulinum toxin procedures. Continued training and mentoring with an experienced instructor are strongly advised to assist with navigating clinical issues that arise in practice over time. It is my sincere hope that this book will enable providers to deliver exceptional care by addressing patients immediate concerns, and through helping them evolve their practice to deliver comprehensive aesthetic care that meets the long-term needs of their patients.

Rebecca Small, MD, FAAFP

Acknowledgments

This book is dedicated to my 17-year-old son, Kaidan Hoang, who showed endless patience while I worked on this project, even when I wrote on our family ski trips and holidays.

I am indebted to my RSMD office staff for their ongoing logistical and administrative assistance. Their support gave me the freedom to write this book and pursue other professional interests, such as teaching and volunteering with the tattoo removal program for at-risk youth. I'm grateful to my patients whose varied aesthetic needs and inquires have continually challenged me to learn and incorporate new techniques, products, and procedures into my practice, and fueled my professional growth over the years.

I want to thank the Division of Plastic and Reconstructive Surgery, the Department of Family and Community Medicine, and the Primary Care Nurse Practitioner Masters Program at UCSF. My teaching experiences with the residents and students have enriched me personally and greatly informed the development of this second edition. Without the trust and participation of the ER, ICU, PACU, and OR UCSF nurses who volunteered as demonstration patients, it would not have been possible to conduct injection Skills Labs for training residents. I would also like to credit Esther Kim, MD, who collaborated with me to develop the first formal outpatient aesthetic curriculum for the plastic surgery residents and wrote the forward for this second edition.

The Natividad Medical Center family medicine residents deserve special recognition. Their interest and enthusiasm for aesthetic procedures led me to develop the first family medicine aesthetics training curriculum in 2008. Special recognition is also due to the primary care providers who participated in my aesthetic courses at the American Academy of Family Physicians' Women's Health, Skin Conditions and Diseases, and Scientific Assembly conferences over the years. Their questions and input further solidified the need for this practical guide series.

It has been a pleasure working with Liana Bauman, the gifted artist who created all of the illustrations for these books. Heather Foltz was the model for many of the illustrated photos in this edition. I appreciate her stamina to hold still during the long sessions required for photo shoots to produce this book.

Special acknowledgements are also due to those at Wolters Kluwer Health who made this book series possible, in particular Brian Brown, Joe Cho, and Ashley Fischer.

Contents

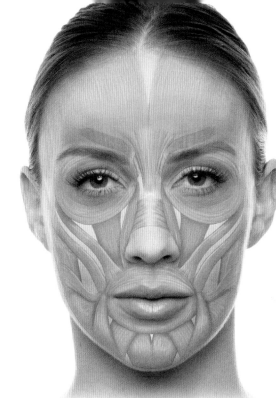

Section 1: Anatomy

Section 2: Introduction and Foundation Concepts

Visit our website for a list of current courses:
RSmdAestheticsTraining.com

Visit our website for a list of current courses:
RSmdAestheticsTraining.com

Section 5: Appendices

Visit our website for a list of current courses:
RSmdAestheticsTraining.com

Section 3: Treatment Areas

Section 4: Cases

Visit our website for a list of current courses:
RSmdAestheticsTraining.com

Section 1

Anatomy

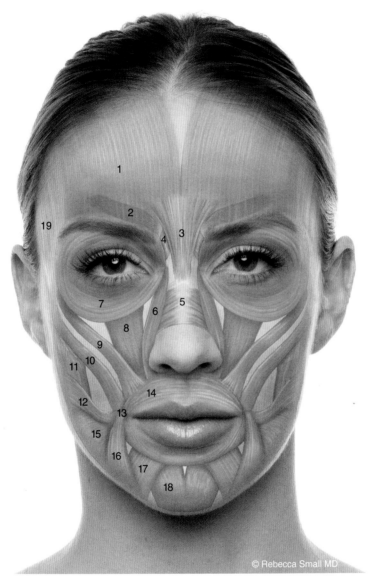

1. Frontalis m.
2. Corrugator supercilii m.
3. Procerus m.
4. Depressor supercilii m.
5. Nasalis m.
6. Levator labii superioris alaeque nasi m.
7. Orbicularis oculi m.
8. Levator labii superioris m.
9. Zygomaticus minor m.
10. Zygomaticus major m.
11. Masseter m.
12. Risorius m.
13. Modiolus
14. Orbicularis oris m.
15. Platysma m.
16. Depressor anguli oris m.
17. Depressor labii inferioris m.
18. Mentalis m.
19. Temporalis m.

FIGURE 1 ● Musculature of the face anterior-posterior. (© Rebecca Small MD.)

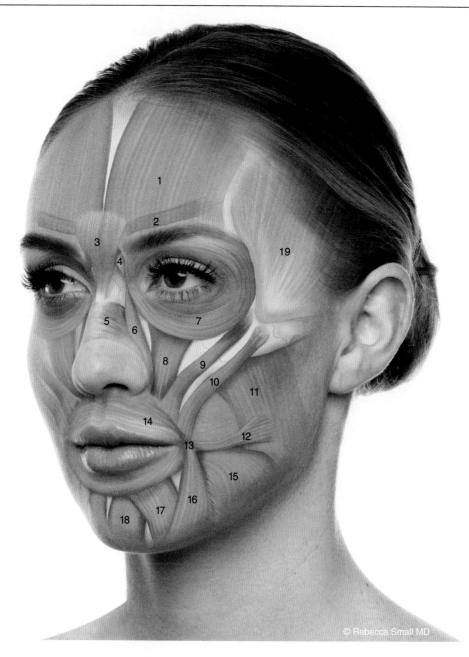

1. Frontalis m.
2. Corrugator supercilii m.
3. Procerus m.
4. Depressor supercilii m.
5. Nasalis m.
6. Levator labii superioris
   alaeque nasi m.
7. Orbicularis oculi m.
8. Levator labii superioris m.
9. Zygomaticus minor m.

10. Zygomaticus major m.
11. Masseter m.
12. Risorius m.
13. Modiolus
14. Orbicularis oris m.
15. Platysma m.
16. Depressor anguli oris m.
17. Depressor labii inferioris m.
18. Mentalis m.
19. Temporalis m.

FIGURE 2 ● Musculature of the face oblique. (© Rebecca Small MD.)

Superficial   **Deep**

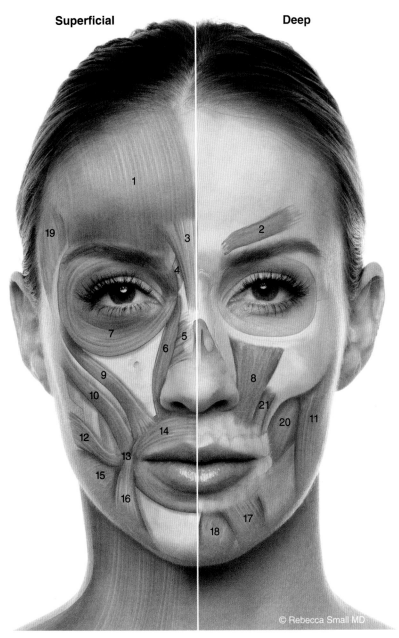

1. Frontalis m.
2. Corrugator supercilii m.
3. Procerus m.
4. Depressor supercilii m.
5. Nasalis m.
6. Levator labii superioris alaeque nasi m.
7. Orbicularis oculi m.
8. Levator labii superioris m.
9. Zygomaticus minor m.
10. Zygomaticus major m.
11. Masseter m.
12. Risorius m.
13. Modiolus
14. Orbicularis oris m.
15. Platysma m.
16. Depressor anguli oris m.
17. Depressor labii inferioris m.
18. Mentalis m.
19. Temporalis m.
20. Buccinator m.
21. Levator anguli oris m.

FIGURE 3 ● Superficial and deep musculature of the face. (© Rebecca Small MD.)

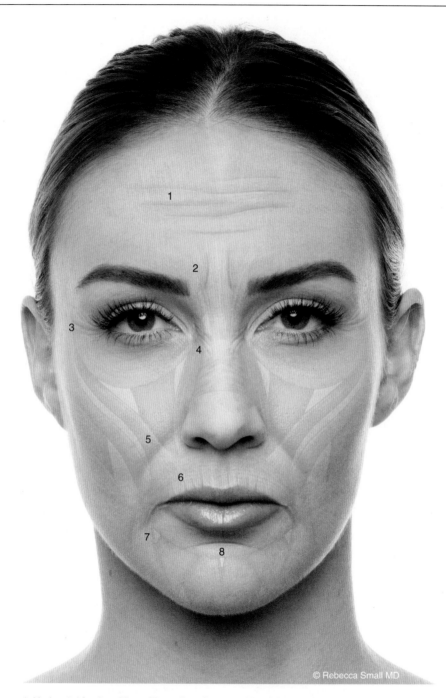

1. Horizontal forehead lines (Frontalis m.)
2. Frown lines (Glabellar complex muscle)
3. Crow's feet (Orbicularis oculi m.)
4. Bunny lines (Nasalis m.)
5. Nasolabial folds (Levator labii superioris alaeque nasi m.)
6. Radial lip lines (Orbicularis oris m.)
7. Marionette lines (Depressor anguli oris m.)
8. Chin line (Mentalis m.)

FIGURE 4 ● Wrinkles and folds of the face anterior-posterior. (© Rebecca Small MD.)

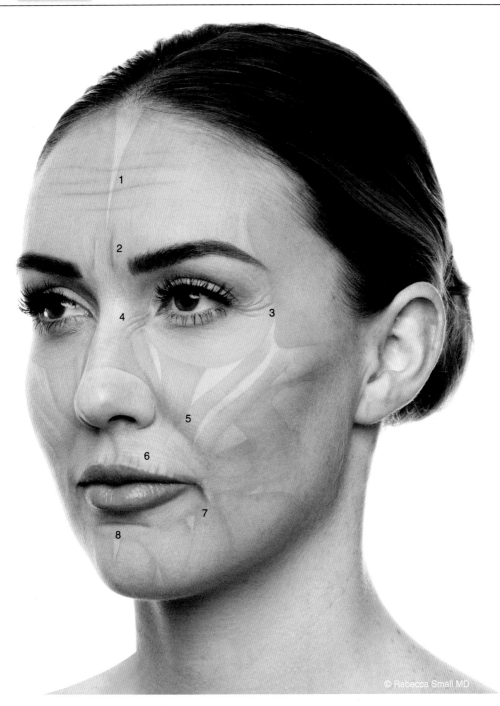

1. Horizontal forehead lines (Frontalis m.)
2. Frown lines (Glabellar complex muscle.)
3. Crow's feet (Orbicularis oculi m.)
4. Bunny lines (Nasalis m.)
5. Nasolabial folds (Levator labii superioris alaeque nasi m.)
6. Radial lip lines (Orbicularis oris m.)
7. Marionette lines (Depressor anguli oris m.)
8. Chin line (Mentalis m.)

FIGURE 5 ● Wrinkles and folds of the face oblique. (© Rebecca Small MD.)

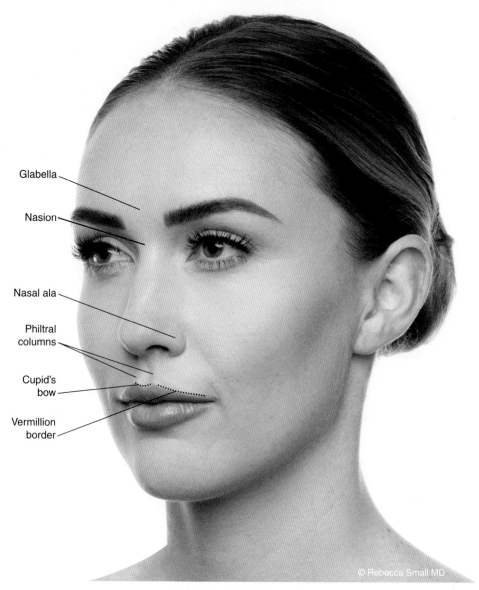

FIGURE 6 ● Facial landmarks. (© Rebecca Small MD.)

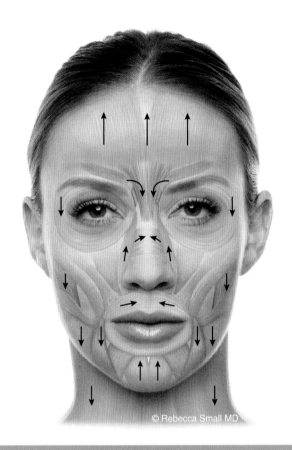

© Rebecca Small MD

TABLE 1

REGION	INDICATION	MUSCLES	ACTIONS
Upper Face	Frown lines	Corrugator supercilii; Procerus and depressor supercilii	Medial eyebrow depressors
	Horizontal forehead lines	Frontalis	Eyebrow levator
	Crow's feet	Lateral orbicularis oculi	Lateral eyebrow depressor
	Eyebrow lift	Superior lateral orbicularis oculi	Superior lateral eyebrow depressor
	Lower eyelid wrinkles	Inferior orbicularis oculi	Eyelid closure
Mid Face	Bunny lines	Nasalis	Nasal sidewalls drawn medially
	Gummy smile	Levator labii superioris alaeque nasi	Central lip levator
Lower Face	Radial lip lines	Orbicularis oris	Lip puckering and mouth closure
	Marionette lines	Depressor anguli oris	Corner of mouth depressor
	Chin line	Mentalis	Chin puckering and lower lip levator
	Square jaw	Masseter	Jaw clenching
	Neck bands	Platysma	Lateral lip and jaw depressor

FIGURE 7 ● Functional anatomy. (© Rebecca Small MD.)
Key: Purple, Depressor muscles; Blue, Levator muscles; Green, Sphincteric muscles.

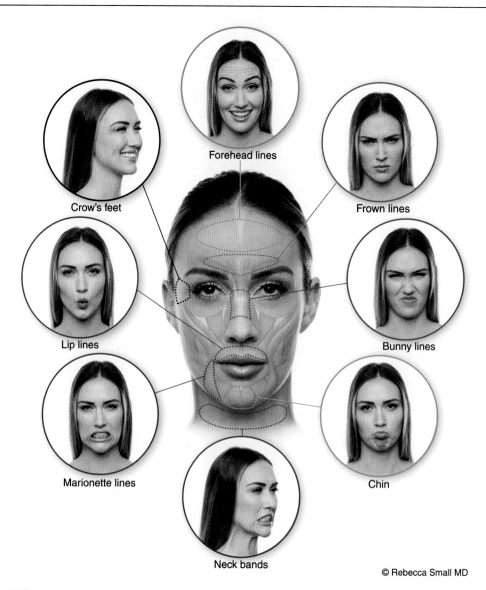

Crow's feet

Forehead lines

Frown lines

Lip lines

Bunny lines

Marionette lines

Chin

Neck bands

© Rebecca Small MD

FIGURE 8 ● Muscles of facial expression. (© Rebecca Small MD.)

TABLE 2

Quick Guide to Botulinum Toxin Dosing for Upper and Mid Face

REGION	INDICATION	MUSCLES TARGETED		TOTAL[a] BTX DOSE(UNITS)
Upper Face	Frown lines		Glabellar complex	20
	Horizontal forehead lines		Frontalis	15
	Crow's feet		Lateral orbicularis oculi	15
	Eyebrow lift		Superior lateral orbicularis oculi	5
	Lower eyelid wrinkles		Inferior preseptal orbicularis oculi	2.5
Mid Face	Bunny lines		Nasalis	3.75
	Gummy smile		Levator labii superioris alaeque nasi	2.5

BTX = onabotulinumtoxinA (Botox®), incobotulinumtoxinA (Xeomin®), and prabotulinumtoxinA (Jeuveau®)

[a]Dose listed is the total starting BTX dose for a given indication (ie., for treatment areas involving bilateral injection this is the combined dose for both sides).

TABLE 3

Quick Guide to Botulinum Toxin Dosing for Lower Face and Neck

REGION	INDICATION	MUSCLES TARGETED		TOTAL[a] BTX DOSE(UNITS)
Lower Face	Lip lines (upper)		Orbicularis oris	5
	Marionette lines		Depressor anguli oris	5
	Chin		Mentalis	7.5
	Angular jaw		Masseter	20
	Anterior neck bands		Anterior platysma	10
	Nefertiti lift		Posterior platysma	15

BTX = onabotulinumtoxinA (Botox®), incobotulinumtoxinA (Xeomin®), and prabotulinumtoxinA (Jeuveau®)

[a]Dose listed is the total starting BTX dose for a given indication (ie., for treatment areas involving bilateral injection this is the combined dose for both sides).

© Rebecca Small MD

Section 2

Introduction and Foundation Concepts

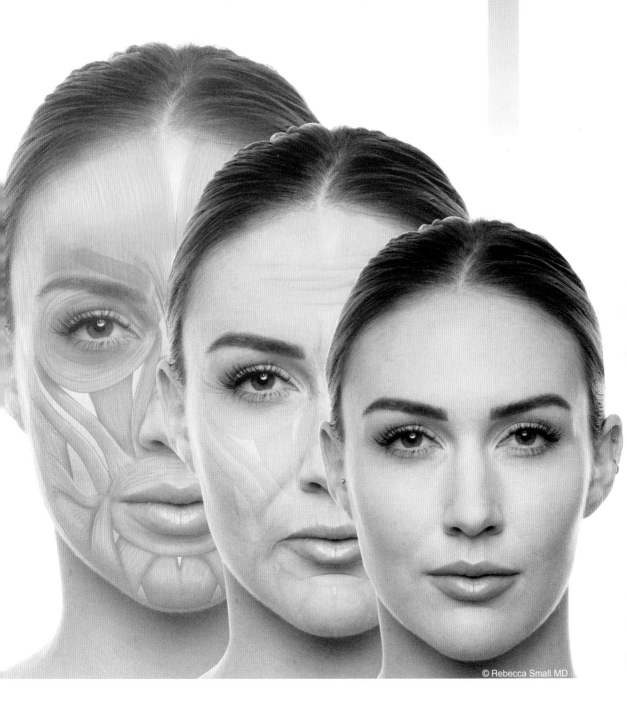

© Rebecca Small MD

11

Administering botulinum toxin injections is an essential skill for physicians and qualified health care providers who wish to incorporate aesthetic medicine into their practice. According to statistics from the American Society of Plastic Surgeons, since its approval for cosmetic use by the U.S. Food and Drug Administration (FDA), botulinum toxin has been the most frequently performed cosmetic procedure for over 20 years with several million treatments performed annually. Success with botulinum toxin procedures and achieving desirable patient results requires knowledge of relevant anatomy and injection skill as well as an appreciation for patients' treatment goals and facial aesthetics.

Facial Aging

Facial aging is a multifactorial process involving changes to skin, fat-pads, muscles and bone. These anatomic changes result in diverse clinical signs of aging such as lax wrinkled skin, loss of volume, descent and flattening of facial contours (Fig. 1).

Wrinkling is a prominent feature of skin aging. Over time, skin naturally thins losing volume and elasticity as dermal collagen, hyaluronic acid, and elastin gradually diminish. This process of dermal atrophy is accelerated and compounded by sun

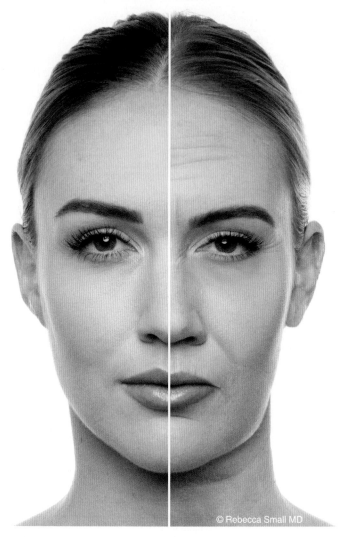

FIGURE 1 ● Half-aged face showing common aging changes.
(© Rebecca Small MD.)

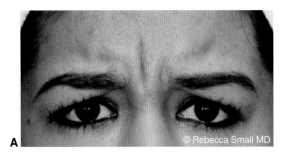

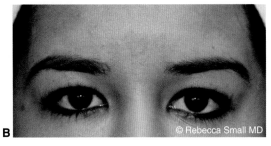

FIGURE 2 ● Younger patient demonstrating dynamic frown lines seen with glabellar complex m. contraction (**A**) and lack of static lines at rest (**B**). (© Rebecca Small MD.)

exposure and other extrinsic factors such as smoking. Hyperdynamic facial musculature also contributes to the formation of visible lines and wrinkles. Initially, lines and wrinkles are seen only during active facial expression such as frowning, laughing, or smiling and are referred to as dynamic lines (Fig. 2A and B). Dynamic lines become etched into skin over time resulting in static lines (Fig. 3A and B) that are present at rest.

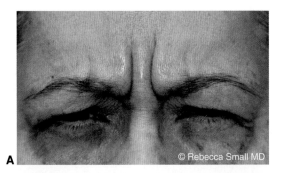

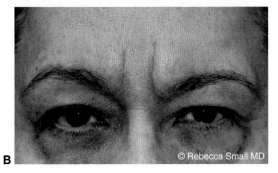

FIGURE 3 ● Older patient demonstrating dynamic frown lines seen with glabellar complex m. contraction (**A**) and static lines at rest (**B**). (© Rebecca Small MD.)

Aged skin also exhibits dyschromia such as mottled pigmentation including solar lentigines, and vascular ectasias including telangiectasias, cherry angiomas, and erythema. Most of these changes are attributable to effects of chronic sun exposure, referred to as photoaging. Benign degenerative changes such as seborrheic keratoses and sebaceous hyperplasia may occur, as well as malignant changes such as basal and squamous cell carcinomas, and melanomas.

In addition to changes seen on the skin surface, many other deep structural changes occur with facial aging. Retaining ligament laxity causes eyebrows to descend and infraorbital hollows (tear troughs) and nasolabial folds to deepen. Descent and atrophy of facial fat pads result in a flattening of the midface and heavier lower face with sagging jowls. Biometric changes such as bone resorption of the orbital rim contribute to infraorbital hollows, loss of alveolar bone and maxillary height lengthen the upper lip and contribute to lip line formation, and loss of mandibular height contributes to chin recession and reduced jawline definition. Overall, an inversion of the youthful facial triangle occurs, whereby high cheekbones and a diminutive lower face change to a widened, square-shaped lower face. Table 1 lists common facial aging changes seen in different decades of life.

TABLE 1

Facial Aging Changes by Decade of Life

Decade	Upper Face	Midface	Lower Face
20s-30s	• Dynamic forehead, glabellar and crow's feet lines • Lower eyelid fine lines	• Dynamic bunny lines • Nasolabial folds	• Dynamic pebbly chin and mental crease
30s-40s	• Forehead, glabellar, and crow's feet lines deepen • Eyebrow descent • Tear troughs	• Malar fat pad descent and malar groove apparent • Nasolabial folds prominent	• Dynamic perioral lines • Oral commissure and marionette lines apparent
40s-50s	• Static glabellar, forehead, and crow's feet lines • Upper eyelid skin laxity • Tear troughs accentuated • Infraorbital fat pad herniation	• Loss of midface volume and anterior projection • Cheek hollows • Nasolabial folds lengthen and deepen	• Lips thin • Static perioral lines • Jawline definition reduced • Jowls apparent • Chin flattened and static mental crease
60s and older	• Upper eyelid laxity worsens with redundant skin folds • Eye aperture reduced • Tear troughs deepen • Infraorbital fat pad herniation worsens	• Static bunny lines • Nasal tip descent • Nasolabial folds worsen	• Lips thin and perioral lines prominent • Oral commissures downturned and marionette lines worsen • Jowls worsen

Anatomy

- Musculature of the face anterior-posterior (Anatomy section, Fig. 1)
- Musculature of the face oblique (Anatomy section, Fig. 2)
- Superficial and deep musculature of the face (Anatomy section, Fig. 3)
- Wrinkles and folds of the face anterior-posterior (Anatomy section, Fig. 4)
- Wrinkles and folds of the face oblique (Anatomy section, Fig. 5)
- Surface anatomy of the face (Anatomy section, Fig. 6)
- Functional anatomy of the face (Anatomy section, Fig. 7)
- Muscles of facial expression (Anatomy section, Fig. 8)

Detailed knowledge of facial anatomy in treatment areas is necessary prior to performing botulinum toxin procedures (Anatomy section, Figs. 1 to 8). Most facial muscles have soft tissue attachments to the skin through the superficial muscular aponeurotic system (SMAS). When facial muscles contract, the overlying skin moves with the muscle causing wrinkles (also called rhytids) to form perpendicular to the direction of muscle contraction. For example, vertical contraction of the frontalis m. forms horizontal forehead lines, and horizontal contraction of the corrugator supercilii muscles form vertical frown lines, commonly referred to as the "elevens."

Functional Anatomy

Facial muscles can be divided into two main functional groups: the levators, which elevate facial structures, and the depressors, which pull structures downward. Figure 7 in the Anatomy section highlights the levator and depressor muscles. Most facial muscles are functionally balanced by opposing muscles. For example, eyebrow position is a balance of the frontalis m. levator function pulling the eyebrows upward against the glabellar complex and orbicularis oculi m. depressor function pulling downward. The position of the corners of the mouth are balanced by the zygomaticus, levator anguli oris, and levator labii superioris alaeque nasi (LLSAN) levator muscles pulling upward against and depressor anguli oris (DAO), depressor inferioris, and facial platysma muscles pulling downward. In youth, levator strength tends to predominate, maintaining an elevated position of soft tissue structures. With age, depressor effects result in an overall downward vector pull and soft tissue descent. When attempting to elevate facial structures such as eyebrows, or enhance a facial contour such as the jawline, treating groups of muscles with botulinum toxin achieves more dramatic improvements than treating single muscles and is often necessary for optimal outcomes.

In addition to aesthetic considerations of wrinkle formation and facial contours, facial musculature is responsible for facial expression, and essential periocular functions such as eye closure and perioral functions such as eating, drinking and articulation. For example, contraction of the orbicularis oculi m. forms crow's feet, changes the position of eyebrows by drawing the lateral eyebrow inferiorly, reduces eye aperture and contributes to blinking. Contraction of the mentalis m. forms the mental crease, skin dimpling, raises the chin, and elevates the lower lip contributing to lip closure. Successful treatment with botulinum toxin requires an appreciation for both aesthetic and functional effects of facial muscles.

Mechanism of Action

Botulinum toxin is a neurotoxin protein derived from the *Clostridium botulinum* bacterium. When small quantities of botulinum toxin are injected into target muscles,

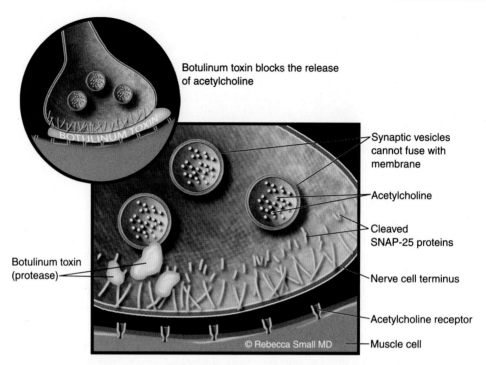

Botulinum toxin blocks the release of acetylcholine

Synaptic vesicles cannot fuse with membrane

Acetylcholine

Cleaved SNAP-25 proteins

Botulinum toxin (protease)

Nerve cell terminus

Acetylcholine receptor

Muscle cell

© Rebecca Small MD

FIGURE 4 ● Botulinum toxin inhibits the release of acetylcholine at the neuromuscular junction. (© Rebecca Small MD.)

localized chemical denervation occurs due to inhibition of acetylcholine release at the neuromuscular junction (Fig. 4). This temporarily reduces muscle contraction and smooths skin wrinkles in the treatment area.

On a cellular level, botulinum toxin A is a protease enzyme that cleaves SNAP-25 (synaptosomal-associated protein, 25 kDa), a docking protein located on the inner surface of the neuronal membrane. This protein is responsible for acetylcholine vesicle fusion at the inner membrane, and once degraded by botulinum toxin, vesicles cannot fuse with the neuronal membrane. Acetylcholine release into the synapse is blocked and neuromuscular signaling inhibited (Fig. 4).

In addition to blocking transmission at the neuromuscular junction, botulinum toxin also blocks acetylcholine transmission at neuroglandular junctions. Inhibition of acetylcholine release in apocrine sweat glands focally reduces perspiration, thereby treating axillary hyperhidrosis.

Botulinum Toxin Products

Clostridium botulinum bacteria produce eight serotypes of botulinum toxin proteins (A, B, Ca, Cb, D, E, F, and G). Botulinum toxin serotype A is the most potent and is used for cosmetic indications. There are five botulinum toxin serotype A products currently approved for cosmetic use in the United States by the FDA: onabotulinumtoxinA (Botox® manufactured by Allergan/AbbVie), abobotulinumtoxinA (Dysport® manufactured by Galderma), incobotulinumtoxinA (Xeomin® manufactured by Merz), prabotulinumtoxinA (Jeuveau® manufactured by Evolus), and daxibotulinumtoxinA (Daxxify® manufactured by ReVance Therapeutics).

TABLE 2

Botulinum Toxin Products

Product	Generic Name	Manufac-turer	Year FDA-Approved	Molecular Weight	Dosing Ratio to Botox	Vial Size	Storage Temperature Unopened
Botox	**Ona**botu-linumtoxinA	AbbVie/Allergan	2002	900 kDa	N/A	100 units	2-8 °C
Dysport	**Abo**botu-linumtoxinA	Galderma/Ipsen	2009	500-900 kDa	2.5:1	300 units	2-8 °C
Xeomin	**Inco**botu-linumtoxinA	Merz	2011	150 kDa	1:1	100 units	20-25 °C or 2-8 °C
Jeuveau	**Pra**botu-linumtoxinA	Evolus	2019	900 kDa	1:1	100 units	2-8 °C
Daxxify	**Daxi**botu-linumtoxinA	ReVance Therapeutics	2022	150 kDa	1:1[a]	100 units	20-25 °C or 2-8 °C

2-8 °C (36-46 °F), refrigerator temperature   © Rebecca Small MD
20-25 °C (68-77 °F), room temperature
[a]1:1 Dosing ratio of daxibotulinumtoxinA is based on data from Carruthers J, Solish N, Humphrey S, et al. Injectable daxibotulinumtoxinA for the treatment of glabellar lines: a phase 2, randomized, dose-ranging, double-blind, multicenter comparison with onabotulinumtoxinA and placebo. *Dermatol Surg.* 2017;43(11):1321-1331.

All botulinumtoxinA products consist of a core active 150 kDa neurotoxin and have varying amounts of complexing proteins called hemaggutinins that surround the core toxin. Some products have no hemagglutinins (eg, Xeomin and Daxxify) while others have many (eg, Botox and Jeuveau) which is reflected in their smaller and larger molecular weights respectively (Table 2). Evidence suggests that complexing proteins have no effect on clinical efficacy, as these proteins dissociate at the time of reconstitution and injection. All currently available botulinum toxin products contain human serum albumin for product stabilization, apart from daxibotulinumtoxinA, which uses a peptide excipient (RTP004).

Dosing Ratios

Dosing ratios are a measure of botulinum toxin clinical efficacy determined by patient response to botulinum toxin products. Xeomin and Jeuveau have a dosing ratio of 1:1 relative to Botox (see Table 2). Dysport has a dosing ratio of 2.5:1 relative to Botox. In other words, 2.5 units of Dysport have a similar clinical effect as 1 unit of Botox. Botulinum toxin products that have 1:1 dosing ratios are abbreviated as BTX in this book and refer to onabotulinumtoxinA (Botox), incobotulinumtoxinA (Xeomin), and prabotulinumtoxinA (Jeuveau). DaxibotulinumtoxinA (Daxxify) also has a dosing ratio of 1:1 relative to Botox. This is demonstrated in a head-to-head trial using 20 units of Botox and 20 units of Daxxify, where no statistically significant differences were found in response or duration of effect in the glabellar muscles for treatment of frown lines (Fig. 8). Due to limited clinical data, daxibotulinumtoxinA is not included with other BTX products and is referenced separately in this book. DaxibotulinumtoxinA (Daxxify) is abbreviated as DBTX. AbobotulinumtoxinA (Dysport) is abbreviated as ABTX.

Botulinum Toxin Units

Botulinum toxin units are a measure of biologic potency and are determined by assays that are proprietary to manufacturers. There is no standardization of units across products and, therefore, products are not interchangeable.

Onset and Duration of Action

All botulinum toxin products have a similar onset of action within 3-5 days and peak effect at 2 weeks (with ABTX onset towards the early part of this range). The duration of action for products currently available with standard dosing (see Standard and High-Dose Botulinum Toxin section) is usually 3.5-4 months in most facial areas. Large muscles such as the masseter and platysma are typically treated with large doses and botulinum toxin effects usually last 6 months; smaller muscles such as the orbicularis oris and nasalis are treated with lower doses and botulinum toxin effects usually last for 2-3 months. Each chapter lists the duration of action for specific treatment areas using standard doses. Duration is affected by several factors including dose, injection technique and patient physiology. Treatments using high doses placed intramuscularly that fully immobilize targeted muscles have longer duration of action (see Duration of Effects and Treatment Intervals in each chapter).

Standard versus High-Dose Botulinum Toxin

Standard botulinum toxin doses are the most common toxin doses used in clinical practice for treatment of a given area, and are usually the same as the FDA-approved or "on-label" dose. For example, the standard and FDA-approved dose for treatment of frown lines is 20 units for BTX products. In some instances, however, the standard dose may differ from the FDA-approved dose. For example, the FDA-approved dose for DBTX is 40 units, which is high-dose. Use of standard versus high doses has implications for duration of action and cost (see High-Dose Toxin chapter). Unless otherwise specified, all references to botulinum toxin doses in this book refer to standard doses.

Patient Selection

Patients with dynamic wrinkles who have minimal to no static component (Fig. 2) demonstrate the most dramatic improvements with botulinum toxin treatments. Patients with static wrinkles also derive benefit from botulinum toxin (Fig. 3), but changes are slower and cumulative, and may require 2-3 consecutive treatments for significant improvements. Combination treatment with dermal fillers is often necessary to achieve optimal results in patients with deep static lines. Discussion of realistic expectations and results during the evaluation and consultation process is essential for patient satisfaction with minimally invasive aesthetic treatments.

Glogau Classification of Photoaging

The Glogau classification is a qualitative scale used to assess severity of facial photoaging, especially with regard to wrinkles (Fig. 5). This baseline measure is usually determined at the time of consultation and used to grossly guide selection and the aggressiveness of aesthetic treatments. In general, Glogau types I to III with mild

Glogau Type	Photoaging	Typical Age	Skin Characteristics	
I	Mild	20s to 30s	Minimal wrinkles No lentigines No keratoses	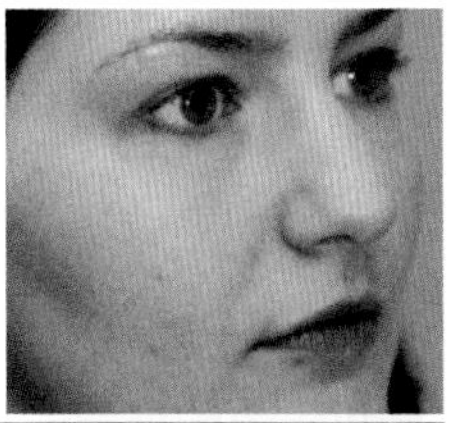
II	Moderate	30s to 40s	Wrinkles in motion Rare, faint lentigines Skin pores prominent Keratoses palpable but not visible	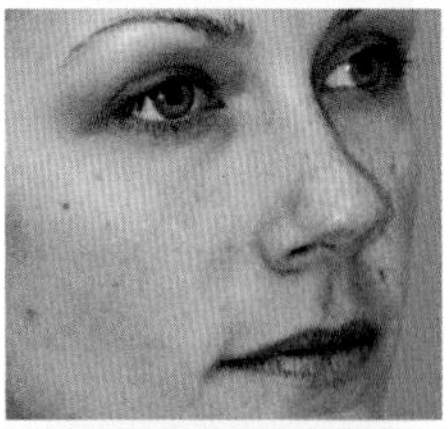
III	Advanced	50s to 60s	Wrinkles at rest Prominent lentigines Telangiectasias Visible keratoses	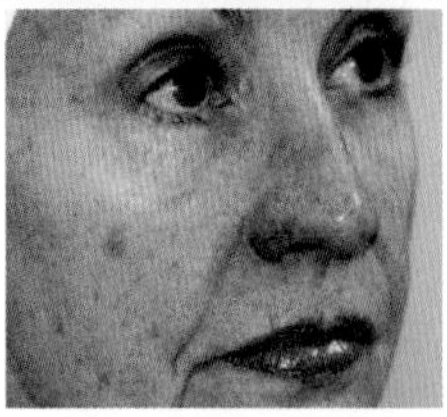
IV	Severe	60s and older	Wrinkles throughout Numerous lentigines Elastosis, coarse pores Yellowish skin color Premalignant lesions and skin malignancies	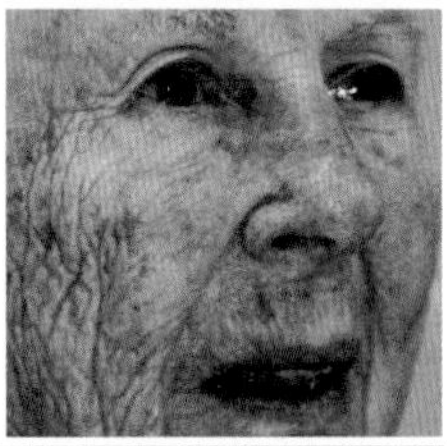

© Rebecca Small MD

FIGURE 5 ● Glogau classification of photoaging. (© Rebecca Small MD.)

to moderate photoaging changes demonstrate skin rejuvenation in response to less aggressive minimally invasive aesthetic treatments such as botulinum toxin, dermal filler injections, and superficial skin resurfacing procedures (Table 4). Glogau type IV patients with severe static wrinkles and laxity often require surgery or aggressive minimally invasive treatments such as deep ablative laser treatments and deep chemical peels for significant wrinkle reduction and skin rejuvenation.

Aesthetic Consultation

Aesthetic consultation is an important part of successfully performing aesthetic treatments and is necessary to determine candidacy for treatment, review procedure details, and set expectations for results. Furthermore, the consultation process provides an opportunity for both providers and patients to assess one another. In addition to evaluating their interaction with a provider, patients assess their experience with the office staff and comfort in the physical space when choosing an aesthetic provider for elective procedures.

Patient Intake

Medical history. As with all medical consultations, standard information is obtained to determine whether patients are good candidates and can safely receive botulinum toxin treatments which includes past medical history, medications, allergies, and surgeries. An example of an aesthetic intake form that may be used during consultation is provided in Appendix 2.

Past cosmetic history. Results from previous minimally invasive procedures and cosmetic surgeries, treatment-related side effects, and satisfaction with outcomes are reviewed. Repeated dissatisfaction with outcomes from prior aesthetic treatments may indicate unrealistic expectations or be a marker for body dysmorphic disorder (BDD). BDD is characterized by a distorted body perception where slight defects in appearance are magnified and patients are hyperaware of these flaws. Patients with unrealistic expectations or BDD are rarely, if ever, satisfied with outcomes from aesthetic procedures, and these are contraindications for treatment.

Social history. Patient motivation for treatment is discussed including upcoming events. If treatments are part of preparation for an upcoming event such as a wedding, success depends on appropriate timing. It is also important to identify occupations for which reduced facial expressivity or reduced articulation may be a concern such as public speaking, and patients whose functionality cannot be compromised, such as musicians who play wind instruments. Patient desire for nondisclosure of treatments to others and tolerance for bruising and down-time can impact the timing of treatments and whether or not to treat. Behaviors that affect facial aging such as smoking and sun exposure are also discussed.

Focused physical examination. Using a handheld mirror, the patient and provider simultaneously examine the areas of concern at rest and with animation. Asymmetries, such as uneven eyebrow height, are pointed out to the patient, noted in the chart, and photographed. Patients are often unaware of asymmetries prior to treatment but may notice them posttreatment and attribute them to the procedure performed.

Functional Assessment. Explaining the functional balance of facial depressor and levator muscles, and synergy of action as they relate to patients' areas of concern is very helpful during consultation. Once patients have an appreciation for muscle actions and how they contribute to their own facial aging issues, patients can better understand the provider approach of treating groups of muscles rather than single muscles to balance facial musculature and enhance results. Ultimately, this broader approach to treatment helps achieve a balanced and natural facial aging pattern over time.

Candidacy for treatment. Based on the history and physical, providers must determine whether or not a patient is a good candidate for minimally invasive treatments. Surgical referral may be necessary for patients with severe laxity and redundant skin folds (Glogau IV), or if minimally invasive treatments will not adequately address patient concerns. Furthermore, if providers cannot meet patient expectations or patients are not a good fit with the practice, care may be declined.

Procedure Terminology

When discussing the specifics of botulinum toxin and other injection procedures, it can be helpful to use nonmedical or "patient friendly" terminology to reduce patient anxiety. Examples of terms used include the following:

Medical Terms	Patient-Friendly Terms
• Toxin	• Natural purified protein
• Paralyzes	• Relaxes
• Pain	• Discomfort

Treatment Plans and Timing

Once candidacy for treatment is determined, an individualized aesthetic treatment plan is created collaboratively with the patient, prioritizing their areas of concern. Treatment options and recommendations are discussed along with anticipated results, realistic expectations, risks of side effects and complications, recovery time, and costs.

Large versus small plans. The decision to present a limited treatment plan versus a larger plan, and whether or not to treat at the time of consultation, depend on the patient's prior experience with botulinum toxin as well as their persona, circumstances affecting timing of treatment, and budget. If patients have limited experience with botulinum toxin and no pressing events, then starting with a small plan that addresses one or two areas of concern is advisable and will gradually build confidence with botulinum toxin treatments and the provider. If, however, the patient has had botulinum toxin treatments regularly for years, is comfortable with all the information presented in the consultation and has few budgetary constraints, then a larger plan can be presented and performed at the visit. Some patients do not desire treatment at the time of consultation but prefer to gather information, contemplate, and decide if they'd like to treat at a future visit. Whether or not patients receive treatment at the consultation or undertake a large or small treatment plan, providers are encouraged to assess the patient's overall facial aesthetics needs and develop a comprehensive plan that is recorded in the chart for future reference.

Short-term and long-term plans. In addition to addressing the patient's immediate concerns, providers are encouraged to have a long-term treatment plan as well. It is important to keep in mind that each procedure performed affects facial aging. Repetitive botulinum toxin treatments strengthen certain muscles and atrophy others, modifying the forces that affect facial regions, essentially sculpting the face over time. Keeping this long-term perspective in mind helps patients achieve a natural pattern of facial aging with repetitive treatments. For example, if a younger person presents with a complaint of horizontal forehead lines, providers may be tempted to treat the frontalis m. only. While treatment of the frontalis m. will reduce forehead lines and satisfy the patient in the short-term, treating only the frontalis m. will unbalance the upper face musculature in the long-term. Upper face depressors will be unopposed, eventually leading to glabellar complex enlargement and eyebrow descent, which creates an unaesthetic appearance as the patient ages. The patient will be unaware of this long-term consequence, and so it is incumbent upon the provider to develop a treatment plan that maintains balance and leads to a natural pattern of aging.

Informed Consent Process

Patients receiving elective aesthetic procedures typically have high expectations of efficacy and low tolerance for side effects. It is advisable to cover all aspects of the informed consent process during consultation, which consists of: (1) discussing the risks, benefits (with emphasis on realistic expectations), alternatives, and complications of the procedure; (2) providing adequate opportunity for all questions to be asked and answered; (3) educating the patient about the nature of their aesthetic issue and procedure details; (4) having the patient sign the consent form; and (5) documenting the informed consent process in the chart. Sample consent forms are included in Appendix 4.

Photodocumentation

Photodocumentation is the use of photography to record and document patient physical findings, procedure results, and complications. While primarily for office purposes, it is also required by some malpractice carriers to document indications for treatment and used for medicolegal purposes. Photographs are typically taken prior to treatment, 2 weeks posttreatment, and if complications occur. Patients are positioned fully upright looking straight ahead and photographs are taken of the full face with close-ups of specific treatment areas from the front, 45°, and 90° angles. Photographs for botulinum toxin treatments are taken with the face at rest and with maximal contraction of muscles in the treatment areas. Consent for photographs is obtained prior to taking photographs and may be included as part of the procedure consent form.

Beauty Norms

Attractiveness and beauty are largely subjective and influenced by social and cultural norms, ethnicity, age, and individual preferences. The most successful, subtle aesthetic treatments do not focus on producing "common, perfect faces," but rather focus on patients' unique facial morphology and enhance particular features that define each individual's face. Treatments ideally maintain congruence with the whole face, achieve balance and symmetry, and are consistent with the patient's underlying age.

Treatment Goals

Optimal outcomes with botulinum toxin treatments result in pleasing aesthetic effects with minimal to no impairment of essential functions in the treatment area. In certain areas of the face, such as the upper face, muscles may be fully immobilized with botulinum toxin without concern for functional impairment, while in other areas, full immobilization can result in severe functional impairment. Each chapter lists Treatment Goals that indicate whether full or partial reduction of muscle contractility is desirable in a given treatment area, which is based on balancing patients' desired aesthetic effects and preserving functionality.

Upper face. In the upper face, muscle contractility is important for facial expressivity but otherwise, there are few essential functions performed by the upper face musculature relative to the lower face. A greater degree of muscle inhibition is typically the goal for treatments in the upper face and patient preferences tend to primarily guide treatment goals. For example, some patients desire complete inhibition of the glabellar complex when treating frown lines, while others desire partial muscle inhibition with retention of some ability to frown. Patient preference is thus the primary determinant for treatment, as functionality is not a significant concern.

Lower face. Lower face muscles perform essential functions of eating, drinking, and speaking. Preserving functionality is the most important consideration when treating this area, more so than aesthetic outcome or patient preference. Therefore, partial inhibition of muscle contraction is the goal for botulinum toxin treatments in the lower face. For example, full immobilization of the upper lip with botulinum toxin treatment of the orbicularis oris m. would achieve the best aesthetic result with regard to reducing lip lines; however, the functional impairment would be intolerable. Therefore, the goal for treatment of the orbicularis oris m. is partial inhibition of contractility to achieve some reduction in upper lip lines while preserving essential oral functionality.

> **Tip**
>
> The goal for botulinum toxin treatments in the lower face is partial inhibition of muscle contraction to ensure essential functions are preserved.

Achieving a Natural Look

Facial aging is characterized by formation of wrinkles throughout the face. A natural pattern of aging can be achieved with botulinum toxin treatments by softening the effects of aging and maintaining balance while avoiding a "treated" look that signals "work" has been done. Ideally, close patient contacts such as coworkers and family should not be able to pinpoint where someone has received treatment but only appreciate that the patient's appearance is improved or that they look rested. A treated look is evident when botulinum toxin treatments result in the following:

Excessive loss of expressivity. Full immobilization of the upper face musculature can result in a "frozen" unnatural look due to loss of expressivity. Some patients associate inability to raise their eyebrows, due to frontalis m. immobility, with loss of expressivity. For most patients, retention of a limited degree of contractility in the frontalis m. and other muscles of the upper face without full immobilization ensures adequate expressivity. Treatment of the glabellar complex may be the exception, where full immobilization is commonly sought by patients and rarely associated with complaints of loss of expressivity.

Lines of demarcation. When focal areas lack wrinkles and surrounding areas have wrinkles, a line of demarcation is apparent, which is not a natural aging pattern. For example, Figure 6 shows a patient that received botulinum toxin treatment in the glabellar complex for frown lines. There is a line of demarcation between the wrinkle free medial forehead where the frontalis m. is noncontractile (due to diffusion of botulinum toxin into the inferior frontalis m. from the glabellar complex), and the surrounding forehead where the frontalis m. has retained contractility and wrinkles. This line of demarcation can be minimized and a natural look achieved by either reducing the dose in the treatment area so that the muscles retain some contractility, or treating the adjacent muscles. In addition to dynamic lines of demarcation, static lines of demarcation can form when botulinum toxin treatments are focused exclusively in one area and performed over long periods of time.

Regional aging differences. Botulinum toxin treatments performed in only one region of the face over time may create an unnatural pattern of facial aging. For example, treatment of the upper face over time without treatment of the lower face can accentuate lower face aging changes relative to the upper face, unbalancing the aging process. A natural look can be achieved by rotating regions of the face treated with botulinum toxin over time so that wrinkling throughout the face is softened, and aging changes in the upper and lower face are consistent.

Compensatory contraction. When several muscles simultaneously engage during a particular facial expression, treating only one muscle with the exclusion of the other muscles can result in compensatory contraction of the untreated muscles. Unnatural

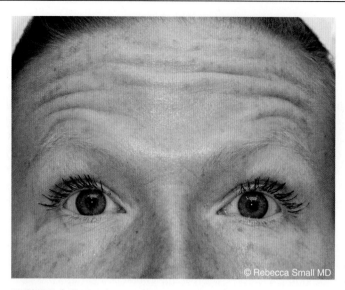

FIGURE 6 ● Botulinum toxin "treated" look visible as peaked lateral eyebrows and a line of demarcation between the immobilized inferomedial frontalis m. and surrounding contractile frontalis muscle. (© Rebecca Small MD.)

contours may become apparent with formation of new wrinkles in the untreated areas creating an unnatural look. For example, excessive lateral eyebrow elevation is an unnatural contour referred to as a peaked eyebrow shape, "quizzical" or "Spock" brow. This is due to botulinum toxin effect in the medial frontalis m. resulting in compensatory contraction of the adjacent lateral frontalis muscle. Figure 6 shows a patient after botulinum toxin treatment of the glabellar complex for frown lines with evidence of peaked "Spock" eyebrows. If this same treatment is performed repetitively over time, new crescent-shaped lines above the lateral eyebrows can form. Bunny lines are another common area where compensatory contraction can result in formation of lines. When treating the orbicularis oculi m. for crows feet or glabellar muscles for frown lines, bunny lines may form on the nose if the nasalis m. is untreated. An understanding of facial muscle contractility in and around treatment areas allows providers to anticipate and, when possible, avoid unnatural compensatory muscle contraction. If compensatory contraction of adjacent muscles does occur, it can be corrected at the 2-week follow-up visit by treating the affected muscle. Each chapter reviews and has treatment recommendations for common follow-up issues to help achieve natural looking patterns of facial aging (see Follow-ups and Management, and Botulinum Toxin Treatment of Other Areas).

Considerations for Specific Populations

Botulinum toxin treatments are individualized and based primarily on patients' unique facial anatomy, musculature and aesthetic preferences. While certain populations may have some common aesthetic concerns and preferences, the focus of aesthetic treatments is the individual patient's needs, which may be very different from perceived norms associated with any ethnic, cultural, age, or gender group. An appreciation for population-specific aesthetic concerns is important, particularly if there are approaches to treatment and injection techniques necessary to address these concerns.

Millennials

Millennials, defined as those born between 1982 and 1996, tend to be early adopters of aesthetic procedures and represent a growing sector of patients seeking botulinum toxin and injectable treatments. Patients in their 20s, such as this population, typically have dynamic wrinkles only and seek botulinum toxin treatment for prevention of static wrinkles, or "prejuvenation," to maintain a youthful appearance. The concept of "paying now" to avoid more costly invasive procedures when they are older often motivates treatment. Botulinum toxin treatments in the upper face are most frequently sought and treatment intervals for these areas can usually be extended to 6 months. Treatments in this population are often less complex compared to older patients, who have the combined challenges of volume loss as well as static lines and other facial aging changes.

Asian Considerations

Certain facial characteristics and unique perceptions of beauty should be taken into account when treating patients of Asian descent or other ethnicities. It is also important to note that Asians do not represent a uniform population, and the following recommendations refer to patients of East Asian and Southeast Asian origin.

Wrinkle formation. Asians may have delayed onset of wrinkle formation and fewer wrinkles relative to Caucasians. As a result, certain facial areas may be less likely to receive treatment such as the upper lip for radial lip lines, and botulinum toxin doses can be as much as 50% lower in Asians than Caucasians. For example, some studies suggest the average dose for treatment of frown lines among Asians is 10 units and forehead lines is 9 units, compared to 20 units and 15 units in Caucasians, respectively.

Facial shape. Anatomically, Asian face shape tends to be wider and more angled at the jaw and flatter in the midface than Caucasian face shape. The broader lower face shape is partly due to greater masseter m. bulk relative to Caucasians and if desired, botulinum toxin can be administered in the masseter muscles to create a narrower, oval face shape (see Masseter chapter). In some cases, botulinum toxin doses can be up to twice that for Caucasians in the masseter m. depending on muscle bulk. Lower face width can be further narrowed by using botulinum toxin in the parotid glands if enlarged. Both Asian women and men commonly seek botulinum toxin facial contouring with botulinum toxin treatment of the masseter muscle.

Eye shape. Asian eyes are typically almond shaped with a smaller palpebral aperture than Caucasians. If desired, a larger, round eye shape can be achieved by placing botulinum toxin in the inferior pretarsal muscle (see Lower Eyelid Wrinkles chapter). However, it is important to note that, in addition to widening eye aperture, botulinum toxin in this muscle can also reduce the pretarsal bulge ("jelly roll"), which some Asians consider to be a beautiful attribute (see Lower Eyelid Wrinkles chapter, Fig. 4-1.) Eye shape and aperture are individual specific, and it is advisable to determine patient preferences prior to treatment to help ensure desired outcomes are achieved.

Eyebrow shape. Eyebrow shape is also highly individualized. While popular with Caucasian patients, high arched eyebrows may be considered harsh by Asians and flatter shaped eyebrows may be preferred. The method used for placement of botulinum toxin in the frontalis can be adapted to achieve these different eyebrow shapes (see Horizontal Forehead Lines chapter).

Darker Skin Type Considerations

Patients with darker skin types, typically of Mediterranean, Asian, Latin, and African descent demonstrate differences in facial aging relative to lighter skin types of Northern European origin. Patients with darker skin types have a delayed onset of wrinkling ranging from 10-20 years later than patients with lighter skin types, due to the photoprotective effect of increased epidermal melanin in darker skin types. Inherent sun protection factor (SPF) can be as high as 13 in black skin versus 3 in white skin. Aging changes commonly seen in darker skin types include hyperpigmentation and changes in the deeper muscle and adipose layers of the face such as midface volume loss, lower eye festoons, and tear troughs rather than superficial lines and skin crepiness seen more commonly in lighter skin types.

Gender Considerations

Certain facial features have been conventionally associated with male and female gender. Examples include a square "male" jaw and high "feminine" arched eyebrows. However, today's facial aesthetics requires a more fluid approach and sensitivity to factors such as cultural, sex, and gender identification. To achieve desired outcomes, providers must develop collaborative treatment plans with patients taking these issues into account, and understand individual preferences in order to meet patient expectations.

Conventional feminine features. The feminine facial contour in youth has more volume in the upper portion of the face compared to the lower portion and is characterized by high cheekbones, slender nose, and small mandible. Well-defined, arched eyebrows that sit at or above the superior orbital rim are also considered feminine features. Injections of botulinum toxin can be used to feminize features where treatment of the glabellar complex elevates eyebrows (see Eyebrow Lift chapter) and treatment of the masseter m. softens jaw angularity (see Masseter chapter). Lips can be defined and volumized using botulinum toxin for eversion (see Lip Lines and Lip Flip chapter) and dermal filler can be used to add volume to the lips and cheekbones (see *A Practical Guide to Dermal Filler Procedures*).

Conventional male features. Conventionally, the male face is more angular and characterized by a square jawline and chin, prominent flat eyebrows that are inferiorly positioned at or just below the superior orbital rim. Masculinization of the face can be achieved by injecting botulinum toxin into the frontalis m. to lower and flatten the brows. Dermal filler can add volume to the jaw and chin to give a more angled appearance (see *A Practical Guide to Dermal Filler Procedures*).

Skin and aging differences. Male skin is thicker and has a higher collagen content with greater density of hair follicles and sebaceous glands compared to female skin. Collagen content reduces at a constant rate for both men and women over time. However, the rate of collagen loss accelerates at menopause due to the rapid decline in estrogen levels and female skin aging changes occur more rapidly, relative to men who experience a gradual decline in testosterone over time. Certain facial areas in men have fewer or no wrinkles relative to women such as perioral lip lines, which is postulated to be due to thicker more sebaceous male skin as well as structural support from upper lip hairs. Furthermore, the male lower face exhibits fewer wrinkles due to regular exfoliation in men who shave, and in those with facial hair, increased protective effect against ultraviolet light from hair. Age-related boney resorptive changes occur in men and women, but the onset is approximately 25 years of age in women compared to 40 years in men.

Advantages of Botulinum Toxin Treatments

- Technically straightforward with short treatment time
- Safe and effective, particularly in the upper third of the face
- Minimal discomfort and bruising
- High patient satisfaction

Disadvantages of Botulinum Toxin Treatments

- Shorter duration of action relative to other cosmetic procedures, although effects are cumulative over time with recurring treatment.

Indications

- All current FDA-approved formulations of botulinum toxin in the United States (Botox, Dysport, Xeomin, Jeuveau, and Daxxify) are approved for the temporary treatment of moderate to severe dynamic frown lines in adults aged 18-65 years. Botox was the first FDA-approved product for treatment of frown lines in 2002, and is approved for treatment of dynamic crow's feet (2013) and forehead lines (2017).
- Botulinum toxin is FDA-approved for the temporary treatment of primary axillary hyperhidrosis (2004), blepharospasm (1989), strabismus (1989), cranial nerve VII disorders (1989), cervical dystonia (2000), upper limb spasticity (2010), and pro-phylaxis for chronic migraine (2010).
- Common off-label cosmetic uses include reduction of other wrinkles in the upper and lower face, neck, and chest, lifting of facial areas, and correction of facial asymmetries.

Contraindications

- Pregnancy or nursing (category C drug in pregnancy)
- Active infection in the treatment area (eg, herpes simplex, pustular acne, cellulitis)
- Hypertrophic or keloidal scarring
- Bleeding abnormality (eg, thrombocytopenia)
- Impaired healing (eg, due to immunosuppression)
- Skin atrophy (eg, chronic oral steroid use, genetic syndromes such as Ehlers-Danlos)
- Active dermatosis in the treatment area (eg, psoriasis, eczema)
- Sensitivity or allergy to constituents of botulinum toxin (including botulinumtoxinA, human albumin, lactose, and sodium succinate)
- Milk allergy with abobotulinumtoxinA products
- Gross motor weakness in the treatment area (eg, due to polio, Bell's palsy)
- Neuromuscular disorder (eg, amyotrophic lateral sclerosis, myasthenia gravis, Lambert Eaton syndrome, and myopathies)
- Inability to actively contract muscles in the treatment area prior to treatment
- Periocular or ocular surgery within the previous 6 months (eg, laser-assisted *in situ* keratomileusis, blepharoplasty)
- Medications that inhibit neuromuscular signaling may potentiate botulinum toxin effects (eg, aminoglycosides, penicillamine, quinine, calcium channel blockers)
- Uncontrolled systemic condition
- Occupation requiring uncompromised facial movement and expression (eg, actors, singers, musicians, public speaking)
- Unrealistic expectations

TABLE 3

Basic, Intermediate and Advanced Botulinum Toxin Treatment Areas

Common Name	Medical Name	Muscles or Target
Basic		
Frown lines	Glabellar rhytids	Glabellar complex: corrugator supercilii, procerus, and depressor supercilii
Crow's feet	Lateral canthal rhytids	Lateral orbital orbicularis oculi
Bunny lines	Nasal rhytids	Nasalis
Excessive underarm perspiration	Axillary hyperhidrosis	Apocrine sweat glands
Intermediate		
Horizontal forehead lines	Frontalis rhytids	Frontalis
Eyebrow lift	Reduction of ptotic eyebrows and dermatochalasis	Superolateral orbital orbicularis oculi
Chin line	Mental crease or labiomental crease	Mentalis
Peau d'orange	Chin dimpling and puckering	Mentalis
Teeth clenching	Masseter hypertrophy	Masseter
Square jaw	Mandible angularity	Masseter
Advanced		
Lower eyelid wrinkles	Infraocular rhytids	Inferior preseptal orbicularis oculi
Lip lines (smoker's or lipstick lines) and lip flip	Perioral rhytids	Orbicularis oris
Marionette lines	Melomental folds or labiomandibular folds	Depressor anguli oris
Downturned corners of the mouth	Oral commissures	Depressor anguli oris
Nasolabial fold	Melolabial folds	Levator labii superioris alequae nasi
Gummy smile	Gingival show	Levator labii superioris alequae nasi
Neck bands	Anterior platysmal bands	Platysma
Nefertiti lift	Posterior platysmal bands	Platysma
Necklace lines	Horizontal neck lines	Platysma
Chest lines	Décolleté lines	Platysma

Basic, Intermediate, and Advanced Treatment Areas

Basic

Treatment of muscles that form wrinkles in the upper face (eg, frown lines and crow's feet) yield the most predictable results, have the greatest efficacy with botulinum toxin treatment, and the fewest reported side effects. Complications associated with treatments in these areas are typically aesthetic rather than functional. These areas are ideal for providers getting started with cosmetic botulinum toxin injections and are referred to as basic or core treatment areas in this book (Table 3). Treatment of axillary hyperhidrosis with botulinum toxin is also a basic area.

Intermediate

Intermediate botulinum toxin areas are the next step in advancement once providers have mastered the core procedures. Some of these treatment areas are more challenging than the basic areas with regard to achieving patient satisfaction (such as horizontal forehead line treatments), and functional complications can occur more frequently (such as chin treatments). If complications arise they usually result from diffusion into adjacent muscles and therefore, have fairly short durations. In general, these are large muscles and there is some margin for error with botulinum toxin placement without adverse-effects.

Advanced

Advanced treatment areas require precise botulinum toxin placement and dosing, have little to no margin for error and aesthetic benefits are subtle, making it more difficult to achieve a high level of patient satisfaction. Botulinum toxin treatment of most muscles in the lower face is considered advanced (eg, lip lines and marionette lines). These muscles serve essential functions of speaking, eating, and drinking and must retain partial functionality, which requires more practiced injection skill. These areas also have a higher frequency of complications, and novice injectors are advised to gain skill and confidence with treating basic and intermediate areas before proceeding to advanced botulinum toxin areas.

Equipment for Botulinum Toxin Reconstitution

- Botulinum toxin 100-unit vial: onabotulinumtoxinA (Botox) or incobotulinumtoxinA (Xeomin) or prabotulinumtoxinA (Jeuveau)
- 5.0-mL syringe
- 0.9% sterile saline 10-mL vial
- 18-gauge, 1.5-in needle

Equipment for Botulinum Toxin Treatment

- Reconstituted botulinum toxin (100 units/4 mL): onabotulinumtoxinA (Botox) or incobotulinumtoxinA (Xeomin) or prabotulinumtoxinA (Jeuveau)
- 1-mL syringe with Luer-Lok™ tip
- 30-gauge, 1.0-in needle
- 30-gauge, 0.5-in needles
- 32-gauge, 0.5-in needles

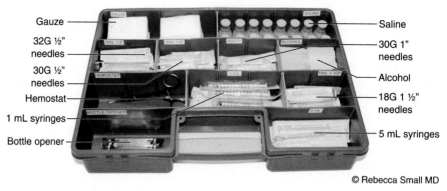

FIGURE 7 ● Equipment for botulinum toxin treatment. (© Rebecca Small MD.)

- 3 × 3-in nonwoven gauze
- Handheld mirror (for consultation)
- Nonsterile gloves
- Alcohol pads
- Ice packs
- Bottle opener (for removal of botulinum toxin vial metal cap to aspirate fluid at the bottom of the vial)
- Hemostat (for loosening tight Luer-Lok connections)
- Soft, white eyeliner pencil or surgical pen (for marking injection sites)

Figure 7 shows an organizational kit for botulinum toxin injection supplies. Syringes with "no-waste" plungers that fill the tip of the syringe and expel all drops of solution are ideal for treatments. Syringes that are 1 mL can affix needles with either Luer-Slip™ tips or Luer-Lok™ tips that screw needles on securely. Syringes that are 0.5 mL or 0.3 mL have needles permanently affixed to them (see Appendix 6, Supply Sources).

Reconstitution Concentrations

Botulinum toxin is supplied as a powder and must be reconstituted into a solution for treatments. There is no standardized concentration of botulinum toxin solution and each manufacturer has a recommendation in their package insert (see Bibliography, Product Package Insert). Small volumes of reconstituted solution are injected for treatments. Providers must be aware of the exact dose associated with each 0.1 mL increment on the injection syringe for accurate dosing of botulinum toxin and are encouraged to use only one concentration of botulinum toxin to reduce variability and achieve predictable outcomes. In addition, selection of the appropriate injection syringe improves accuracy with small volumes.

Reconstitution of BTX (Botox, Xeomin, and Jeuveau) 100-unit vial with commonly used diluent volumes, resultant doses per 0.1 mL, and recommended injection syringes are shown below:

Diluent Volume Added to 100-Unit Vial of BTX (mL)	Dose per 0.1 mL Reconstituted BTX Solution (units)	Injection Syringe (mL)
1.0	10	0.3 or 0.5
2.0	5	0.3 or 0.5
2.5	4	0.3 or 0.5
4.0	2.5	1.0

Reconstitution of Dysport 300-unit vial with commonly used diluent volumes and resultant doses per 0.1 mL are shown in Appendix 1, Table 2B. Reconstitution of high-dose botulinum toxin (eg, Daxxify) is shown in the High-Dose Toxin chapter.

 Tip

In this book, 100 units BTX is reconstituted with 4-mL saline:
- Injections are performed with 1-mL syringe
- Each 0.1 mL of reconstituted solution has 2.5 units BTX

Reconstitution Method

Reconstitution of BTX (Botox, Xeomin, and Jeuveau) is described below and used throughout this book. Sterile nonpreserved saline (recommended by manufacturers) or preserved bacteriostatic saline with benzyl alcohol may be used as the diluent. Solutions reconstituted with preserved saline are associated with less injection discomfort due to higher pH; both preserved and nonpreserved solutions have equivalent efficacy. The author reconstitutes a 100-unit vial of BTX with 4-mL saline (100 units/4 mL) as follows:
- Using an 18-gauge needle with a 5.0-mL syringe, draw up 4.0 mL of 0.9% sterile saline
- Insert the needle at a 45° angle into a 100-unit BTX vial and inject saline slowly, maintaining upward plunger pressure so that the diluent runs down the sides of the vial
- Gently swirl the reconstituted BTX vial, record the date and time of reconstitution on the vial, and store in the refrigerator 2 to 8 °C (36-46 °F)

While studies have shown that reconstituting rapidly with vigorous shaking and foaming of the product does not appear to result in loss of clinical effect, proteins are fragile and it's advisable to use gentle handling practices with botulinum toxin.

Reconstitution methods for high-dose botulinum toxin treatments are reviewed in High-Dose Toxin chapter and for ABTX in Appendix 1, Table 2.

Conversion Tables for Injection Volumes

Once botulinum toxin has been reconstituted, the appropriate volume of botulinum toxin solution corresponding to the treatment dose is aspirated from the vial. To help ensure accuracy of injection volumes, the following tables are provided that convert botulinum toxin treatment doses (units) to injection volumes (mL) based on different reconstitution concentrations:
- BTX reconstituted with 4-mL saline diluent, which is used in this book (Appendix 1, Table 1A).
- BTX reconstituted with 2.5-mL, 2-mL and 1-mL saline diluent (Appendix 1, Tables 1B to 1D).

Diffusion

While botulinum toxin efficacy and duration are primarily based on the number of units injected and technique used, diffusion of botulinum toxin also has implications for treatment effects. Diffusion is influenced by reconstitution concentration, where less concentrated solutions (using larger diluent volumes) result in a greater area of diffusion. When the same number of units are injected, the field effect around each injection site from a less concentrated solution is greater than the field effect from a more concentrated solution. For example, a 100-unit vial of BTX reconstituted with 5 mL results in approximately a 1 cm radius of diffusion from an injection site, whereas reconstitution with 1 mL results in a 50% smaller area of diffusion. Reconstitution volumes up to 5 mL do not increase the rate of adverse effects, however, excessive dilution volumes of 10 mL or more are associated with increased complications due to undesired effects in adjacent muscles from greater diffusion. Selection of the volume used for reconstitution is largely based on provider preference for diffusion characteristics and ease of dose calculations.

Handling and Storage

Botox, Jeuveau, and Dysport are shipped frozen on dry ice and prior to reconstitution are stored in the refrigerator at a temperature of 2-8 °C (36-46 °F). Xeomin and Daxxify are shipped at room temperature and prior to reconstitution may be stored either in the refrigerator or at room temperature 20-25 °C (68-77 °F). Botulinum toxin products have shelf lives of 24-36 months prior to reconstitution, depending on the manufacturer. While manufacturers recommend using botulinum toxin within 24 hours of reconstitution, the American Society for Plastic Surgery Botox Consensus Panel recommends using botulinum toxin within 6 weeks after reconstitution and notes no loss of potency or sterility during that time.

Preprocedure Checklist

- Perform an aesthetic consultation and obtain informed consent.
- Take pretreatment photographs with the patient actively contracting the muscles in the intended treatment area and with the muscles at rest.
- Document and discuss any notable asymmetries before treatment.
- Minimize bruising by discontinuation of aspirin, turmeric, fish oil, vitamin E, ginkgo, evening primrose oil, garlic, feverfew, ginseng and any other supplements associated with anticoagulation for 2 weeks. Discontinue other nonsteroidal anti-inflammatory medications and alcohol consumption 2 days before treatment.
- For hyperhidrosis treatment, discontinue antiperspirant use 24 hours before treatment and see Hyperhidrosis chapter for other preprocedure steps.

Procedure

1. Reconstitute the botulinum toxin vial with saline according to the desired reconstitution concentration.
2. Position the patient comfortably in a reclined position at about 65° angle.
3. Identify the Safety Zone for treatment, which is the recommended region within which injections are administered, using the Safety Zone illustration in each chapter.
4. Locate the target muscles for botulinum toxin injection within the Safety Zone by instructing the patient to contract the relevant muscles using specific facial expressions as outlined in each chapter.
5. Identify the botulinum toxin injection sites and botulinum toxin starting doses for the treatment area using the Overview of Injection Sites and Doses figure in each chapter.

6. Instruct the patient to close their eyes during the procedure to reduce patient movement.
7. Cleanse the treatment areas with alcohol prior to injection and allow alcohol to dry.
8. Inject the target muscles using the techniques for the specific treatment area outlined in each chapter.
9. Compress sites after performing injections to reduce bruising.

 Tip

Confining treatment to the Safety Zone area maximizes efficacy and reduces the risk of adverse effects.

Anesthesia

Anesthesia is not typically required for botulinum toxin treatments. If necessary, ice or a topical anesthetic such as benzocaine 20%:lidocaine 6%:tetracaine 4% (BLT) cream or ointment may be applied for 15-20 minutes prior to treatment. Effects of topical anesthetics are enhanced by occluding the product under plastic wrap once applied to the skin.

Product	Composition	Source
• L-M-X	• Lidocaine 4%-5%	• Over-the-counter
• EMLA	• Lidocaine 2.5%: prilocaine 2.5%	• Prescription
• BLT	• Benzocaine 20%: lidocaine 6%: tetracaine 4%	• Compounded by a pharmacy

See Appendix 6, Supply Sources.

BLT is a potent and fast-acting topical anesthetic and is preferred for use by the author. It is used in-office, with a maximum dose of 0.5 g applied topically. Occlusion under plastic wrap is not necessary with BLT due to its potency. While maximal application time is 45 minutes, 15-20 minutes is usually sufficient for an adequate anesthetic effect with BLT.

 Tip

For quick reference, summary tables of botulinum toxin treatment doses are provided:

• Upper face BTX doses (Anatomy section, Table 2)
• Lower face BTX doses (Anatomy section, Table 3)
• Upper and lower face ABTX doses (Appendix 1, Table 2).

Botulinum Toxin Treatment Doses

• Botulinum toxin treatment doses are primarily determined by muscle mass, where large muscles require greater doses. Large muscle mass is associated with hypertrophied muscles, male gender, and large body size. Hypertrophied muscles tend to bulge visibly with contraction and are palpably larger and firmer than average muscles. Men typically have larger muscles than women and, therefore, require greater botulinum toxin doses to achieve equivalent results (see Starting Doses listed in each chapter). Tall individuals have proportionally larger muscles; for example, a woman 5'10" or taller typically requires a greater dose than a woman 5' or shorter.

- Botulinum toxin doses referenced in this book refer to standard doses (see Standard and High-Dose Botulinum Toxin) and recommended starting doses for treatment areas are listed in each chapter (see Overview of Injection Sites figures)
- It is advisable to limit the total treatment dose for all areas to less than 100 units BTX in one visit when getting started with botulinum toxin treatments. This is particularly important when treating large muscles such as the masseter and platysma, multiple muscles, axillary hyperhidrosis, and when performing high-dose treatments.

 Tip

Maximum combined botulinum toxin dose recommended for all treatments in a single session is 100 units BTX for providers just getting started, and may be greater than 100 units BTX per session for experienced providers.

General Injection Techniques

- The target for all botulinum toxin treatments described in this book is muscles, apart from axillary hyperhidrosis. The target for axillary hyperhidrosis is apocrine sweat glands located in the dermis.
- In areas where the skin is thin, muscles are superficially located and subdermal injection adequately delivers botulinum toxin to the target muscle. In other areas, deeper intramuscular injection technique is required. Procedure Overview in each chapter lists the appropriate injection depth for a given treatment area.
- The needle is inserted into the area of maximal muscle contraction, which is visible as a "hill" or "ridge" of muscle.
- Botulinum toxin is typically injected as a bolus at the desired depth where the needle tip is inserted, or in a linear thread as the needle is withdrawn, and flows very easily with minimal plunger pressure. If resistance is encountered, fully withdraw the needle and reinsert.
- Avoid intravascular injection. Intravascular injection is apparent when the surrounding skin blanches during injection. If this occurs, withdraw the needle partially from the blanched site, reposition, and inject.
- Avoid hitting the periosteum, particularly with frontalis m. treatments, as touching bone is painful and dulls the needle.
- Small gauge needles (eg, 30 gauge and 32 gauge) are used for injection to minimize discomfort and bruising, but dull quickly. Consider changing needles after six injections or when more force is required to puncture the skin, to minimize discomfort and improve injector control.
- After injecting, the site may be compressed with gauze to reduce discomfort, bleeding, and bruising. When treating around the eye, compression is directed away from the eye. When treating the neck, pinching a bruise is often necessary as there are no hard structures to compress against.
- If bleeding occurs, achieve hemostasis before proceeding to subsequent injection sites to reduce the risk of bruising.
- Avoid vigorous massage of the area or excessive exercise after treatment to minimize undesired migration of botulinum toxin to adjacent muscles.

Tip

Depth of botulinum toxin injections is site specific and can be visually determined as follows:

- Intradermal injections are visible as a wheal with dimpled skin (eg, treatment of axillary hyperhidrosis)
- Subdermal injections are visible as a wheal without dimpled skin (eg, treatment of crow's feet)
- Intramuscular injections are visible as a subtle wheal without dimpled skin or as generalized edema in the injection area (eg, treatment of frown lines)

Aftercare

On the day of treatment, patients are instructed to avoid lying down for 4 hours immediately after treatment, manipulating the treated area (eg, a facial or massage), and activities that can cause facial flushing (eg, application of heat to the face, alcohol consumption, vigorous exercise, and tanning) to reduce the likelihood of product migration and risk of side effects. If bruising or swelling occurs, a soft ice pack may be applied for 10-15 minutes to each bruise site, every 1-2 hours until improved. Intense pulsed light (IPL) and vascular laser treatments can significantly hasten bruise resolution. While there is little evidence in the literature to support or refute most aftercare practices, some data support minimizing the application of ice after treatment as cold temperatures decrease cellular uptake of botulinum toxin and may reduce efficacy. In addition, limited data suggest active facial expression within 4 hours of botulinum toxin treatment may increase the rapidity of onset of effects by 1-2 days.

Results and Follow-Up

- Treated muscles typically demonstrate partial reduction in function within 3-5 days after botulinum toxin treatment, with maximal reduction 2 weeks after treatment.
- Effects are most dramatic for treatment of dynamic lines. Static lines are slower to respond, and typically require two to three consecutive treatments for noticeable improvements, depending on severity. Combination treatment with other minimally invasive aesthetic procedures such as dermal fillers or resurfacing procedures helps achieve optimal results for areas with static lines (see Combination Therapies).
- A follow-up visit is scheduled 2 weeks after the initial treatment to assess outcomes and refine results if needed. Anticipated results for treatment areas are reviewed in the Results section of each chapter.
- If desired reduction of muscle function is not achieved in the treatment area, a touch-up procedure may be performed at the 2 week follow-up visit. The botulinum toxin touch-up dose varies according to the degree of movement remaining in the target muscles, patient preference, and the need to preserve essential functions (see individual chapters for recommended touch-up doses). The treatment area is reassessed 2 weeks after the touch-up procedure. Photos are taken at each visit to record progress.
- The optimal dose of botulinum toxin for treatment is determined to be the initial dose plus the touch-up dose. This total dose may be used at the patient's subsequent treatment.
- Results of botulinum toxin treatments in the lower face are subtle, relative to changes seen in the upper face. Patients may be able to appreciate pre- and posttreatment improvements in dynamic lines in the lower face if shown how to assess muscle contractility with animation. In addition to a pleasing aesthetic effect, a desirable result in the lower face has no impairment of essential oral functions such as eating, drinking, and speaking.

- Muscle function in the treatment area gradually returns 3½-4 months after treatment for most muscles and is affected by the botulinum toxin dose and patient's physiology.
- Subsequent treatments are recommended when muscle function in the treated area recurs, prior to facial lines or undesired muscle functions returning to their pretreatment state. Anticipated duration of effects and recommended intervals for treatment are reviewed in Duration of Effects and Treatment Intervals in each chapter.

 Tip

Results from botulinum toxin treatments are fully evident 2 weeks after treatment and typically last 3½-4 months, though this may vary based on the area treated and patient-specific factors.

 Tip

Consistent retreatment of the target muscles over time may extend intervals between treatments, likely resulting from muscle atrophy.

Learning the Techniques

- Marking the Safety Zone and injection sites with a soft, white eyeliner pencil or surgical marker before treatment can help with locating the target muscles for treatment and define the area within which botulinum toxin can be safely administered. Each chapter has a Safety Zone and Overview of Injection Sites figure for reference.
- It is advisable to start with conservative botulinum toxin doses and each chapter has recommended starting doses for a given treatment area.
- Performing initial treatments on staff and family provides valuable feedback and close observation of botulinum toxin effects.
- Touch-up procedures performed 2 weeks after initial treatment are helpful for improving injector technique and dosing.
- Detailed documentation of minor side effects improves injector skill and technique over time as well as patient satisfaction with treatments.
- Consider receiving a treatment to gain personal knowledge about botulinum toxin procedures.

Complications and Management

Complications and adverse reactions can be categorized as injection-related or botulinum toxin–related issues. Most complications with botulinum toxin treatments are injection related, minor, and resolve spontaneously. Complications associated with each treatment area and suggestions for management are discussed in individual chapters. For example, blepharoptosis listed here is reviewed in the Frown Lines chapter. The Bibliography contains references for further reading in Complications and Management and in the respective sections for each treatment area.

Injection-Related Complications

- Pain
- Bruising
- Erythema

- Edema
- Tenderness
- Headache
- Jaw pain
- Infection
- Numbness or dysesthesia
- Anxiety
- Vasovagal episode and loss of consciousness

Pain with botulinum toxin injections is minimal as small-gauge needles are used for treatment. If necessary, injection pain can be reduced using ice or topical anesthetics. While topical anesthetic may be used in areas of high sensitivity such as bunny lines and the upper lip, extensive pretreatment use of topical anesthetics can increase visit times and is not necessary.

Bruising is commonly seen with botulinum toxin injections, particularly treatment of crow's feet. Bruises can range in size from pinpoint needle insertion marks to quarter-sized ecchymoses or, rarely, hematomas. The time for resolution of a bruise depends on the patients' physiology and the size of the bruise, where larger bruises can be visible for up to 2 weeks. Several suggestions for bruise prevention are listed in the Preprocedure Checklist. Immediate application of ice and pressure to a bruise can minimize bruise formation. Vascular lasers such as the 532 nm, 595 nm pulsed dye, and intense pulsed light (IPL) can accelerate bruise resolution dramatically. Ice may also be applied to bruises after treatment to facilitate resolution. Bruises may be concealed using makeup with appropriate counter colors (eg, yellow cancels red, peach cancels blue, and lilac cancels yellow).

Erythema, **edema** and mild injection site **tenderness** occur with almost all injections and usually resolve within a few hours after treatment. Firm compression of injection sites immediately after injection can effectively reduce edema, particularly wheals on the forehead. Icing is not typically used for these issues.

Headache can occur with upper face injections, and **jaw pain** can occur with masseter m. injections. While botulinum toxin is a treatment for headaches and jaw pain, patients with pain syndromes in these areas are predisposed to exacerbation immediately postprocedure. Most headaches are mild (5% incidence) and resolve within a few days after treatment without medication. There are reports of idiosyncratic severe headaches (1% incidence) lasting 2-4 weeks. Headaches occur more often with botulinum toxin treatment of the frown and forehead relative to other treatment areas. Nonsteroidal anti-inflammatory medications are usually adequate for management of headaches and jaw pain. If patients are in acute pain preprocedure when they present for treatment, it is advisable to postpone treatment until they are pain free.

Infection is rare with botulinum toxin injections but can occur with any procedure that breaches the skin barrier. The most common etiologies are bacterial or reactivation of herpes simplex (eg, cold sores) or herpes zoster (ie, shingles). Prolonged **pain, tenderness,** and **erythema** of more than a few days' duration can signal infection and necessitate evaluation and infection-specific treatment.

Numbness or **dysesthesia** in the treatment area is extremely rare and could result from nerve injury with injections.

Anxiety with injection procedures is common. Most patients have mild procedural anxiety, which can be reduced by ensuring that injection equipment is not visible during treatment and can be managed during the procedure with breathing techniques. Rarely, patients with more severe anxiety may require preprocedural medications (eg, tramadol 50 mg, 1 tablet 30 minutes prior to procedure).

Vasovagal episodes with **loss of consciousness** are possible, and it is advisable for offices to have emergency protocols and emergency medications (such as ammonium carbonate smelling salts) readily available when performing injection procedures.

 Tip

The most common injection-related complication is bruising. The risk of bruising can be reduced with preprocedure preventative measures.

Botulinum Toxin–Related Complications

- Localized burning or stinging pain during injection
- Blepharoptosis (droopy eyelid)
- Eyebrow ptosis (droopy eyebrow)
- Ectropion of the lower eyelid (eyelid margin eversion)
- Lagophthalmos (incomplete eyelid closure)
- Xerophthalmia (dry eyes)
- Epiphora (excess tearing)
- Diplopia (double vision)
- Impaired blink reflex
- Photophobia (light sensitivity)
- Globe trauma
- Infraorbital festoons (eye bags)
- Lip ptosis (lip droop) with resultant smile asymmetry
- Oral incompetence with resultant drooling and impaired speaking, eating, and drinking
- Cheek flaccidity
- Dysarthria (difficulty articulating)
- Dysphagia (difficulty swallowing) with nasogastric tube placement in severe cases and aspiration
- Dysphonia (hoarseness)
- Neck weakness
- Facial asymmetry
- Inadequate reduction of wrinkles or lack of intended effect in the treatment area
- Worsening wrinkles in areas adjacent to the treatment area
- Weakened muscles adjacent to the treatment area with undesired aesthetic or functional change
- Antibodies against botulinum toxin
- Allergic and immediate hypersensitivity reactions with urticaria, edema, and in extreme cases anaphylaxis and death
- Systemic botulism-like effects with diplopia, blurred vision, bilateral eyelid ptosis, dry mouth, dysphagia, asthenia (generalized muscle weakness), urinary incontinence, dyspnea (respiratory difficulties), respiratory failure, and death

Adverse effects and complications associated with botulinum toxin itself are typically mild and self-limited. While major complications have been reported; they are extremely rare and occur more often with large doses used for therapeutic indications (eg, muscle spasticity associated with cerebral palsy) rather than cosmetic applications of botulinum toxin. Safety data are greatest for botulinum toxin products that have been in clinical use for the longest period of time such as onabotulinumtoxinA (Botox), abobotulinumtoxinA (Dysport), and incobotulinumtoxinA (Xeomin).

Localized burning or stinging pain can be reduced by using bacteriostatic preserved saline for reconstitution of botulinum toxin.

Weakening of muscles adjacent to the treatment area account for most of the adverse events and complications seen with botulinum toxin treatments. Weakening of adjacent muscles results from diffusion or incorrect placement of botulinum toxin injections and can cause undesired aesthetic effects and functional changes in these muscles. Diffusion can occur horizontally and vertically, affecting muscles lateral, superficial or deep to the targeted muscle. For example, when treating the mentalis m. lateral diffusion can affect the depressor labii inferioris m., and when treating neck bands deep diffusion can affect the strap muscles. Large reconstitution volumes, greater than standardly used in clinical practice (eg, 10 mL of diluent in 100 units BTX), are associated with greater diffusion and can increase risks of complications such as eyelid ptosis from glabellar complex injections. However, lower reconstitution volumes (eg, 5 mL or less) that are standardly used, are not associated with increased risks of complications. Adjacent muscle involvement is more common in the lower face, where small muscles are closely approximated and interdigitate with one another, compared to the upper face.

The duration of adverse effects in adjacent muscles is greatest when botulinum toxin is directly injected rather than diffuses into an unintended muscle. Adverse effects from direct injection typically last 3½-4 months, depending on the treatment area, whereas adverse effects due to diffusion have a shorter duration, typically in the order of weeks. Some adverse effects can be diminished with botulinum toxin treatment of muscles that antagonize the affected muscles. For example, lateral eyebrow ptosis may be improved with an eyebrow lift procedure. However, there are no corrective treatments for most complications associated with botulinum toxin effects in adjacent muscles and adverse effects resolve spontaneously as botulinum toxin effects diminish.

Antibody formation against botulinum toxin can render treatments ineffective but is a very rare occurrence with botulinum toxin used for cosmetic treatments. Several studies report a 0.5-1% incidence of antibody formation to cosmetic botulinum toxin. If patients are nonresponsive to botulinum toxin treatment, consider using a different botulinum toxin product at the subsequent treatment, and extending the treatment interval to 6 months. If nonresponse persists, perform serologic testing for botulinum toxin antibodies to determine if immunity is the etiology. Note that partial response to botulinum toxin with reduced muscle contractility is not indicative of antibody formation and is more likely associated with dosing, technique, or compensatory contraction of adjacent muscles.

Allergic and immediate hypersensitivity reactions are extremely rare, occur more often with therapeutic botulinum toxin applications, and include prolonged edema, urticaria, anaphylaxis and death. A case of anaphylaxis leading to death was reported from treatment with 100 units Botox in the neck for cervical dystonia. Use of standard emergency protocols and medications such as epinephrine and methyl-prednisolone, and appropriate urgent referral are advised when indicated.

Systemic botulism-like effects related to distant spread of botulinum toxin remote from the injection site, have been reported with large doses of botulinum toxin used for therapeutic applications such as muscle spasticity. Symptoms include dry mouth, diplopia, pupil dilation, bilateral eyelid ptosis, diminished gag reflex, dysphagia, dysarthria, dysphonia, descending paralysis with diaphragmatic paralysis, and respiratory failure. There are case reports of death in patients receiving botulinum toxin for therapeutic indications in patients with compromised baseline respiratory status (eg, children receiving 6-32 units/kg of Botox for treatment of muscle spasticity associated with cerebral palsy). There are extremely rare case reports of systemic botulism-like effects in patients receiving botulinum toxin for cosmetic indications. For example, a patient who incorrectly received 300 units Botox for axillary hyperhidrosis presented with signs of botulism including dysphagia, choking at night, diplopia, and generalized weakness.

Severe complications including hypersensitivity anaphylactic reactions and systemic botulism-like effects can be medical emergencies requiring emergent care and consultation with appropriate medical specialists. Severe botulinum toxin complications can be managed with a botulinum toxin reversal agent, pyridostigmine (Mestinon) 60 mg IV/PO TID, an acetylcholinesterase inhibitor routinely used for myasthenia gravis. Cholinergic side effects of this medication include increased gastric motility, salivation, and urination. Heptavalent botulism antitoxin contains neutralizing antibodies to botulinum toxin and is also indicated for treatment of systemic botulism-like effects. Relative to pyridostigmine, it is less readily available and may have limited utility as it only neutralizes circulating botulinum toxin and does not reverse preexisting botulism systemic effects. It is important to note that life-threatening complications have not been reported with cosmetic use of botulinum toxin up to 100 units BTX in a given visit.

In summary, the risk of adverse effects and complications related to botulinum toxin injection can be reduced with detailed knowledge of anatomy in the treatment area, accurate identification of injection sites, and precise injection technique.

 Tip

The most common botulinum toxin-related complication is weakening of muscles adjacent to the treatment area. The risk of this adverse-effect is reduced when injections are placed in the defined Safety Zones and as injector skill improves.

Treatment of Multiple Muscles

Botulinum toxin treatment of multiple muscles in different regions, such as the upper face and lower face, can be readily combined during one treatment session. For example, treatment of frown lines in the upper face and depressor anguli oris m. (DAO) in the lower face may be treated concomitantly.

Treatment of multiple muscles within one region can also be combined in one session; however, there is greater potential for adverse effects and more careful consideration of functional impairment and balancing muscle contractility is necessary. Factors to consider when treating multiple muscles within one region are discussed below:

Upper face. Multiple muscles are often concomitantly treated in the upper face, particularly when balancing levator and depressor m. functions to elevate eyebrows.

For example, the glabellar complex and orbicularis oculi muscles are routinely treated concomitantly, shifting the depressor - levator balance in the upper face to elevate eyebrows. Some patients have concerns regarding loss of expressivity when all upper face muscles are concomitantly treated. In these cases, providers may rotate treatment areas over time rather than treating all muscles in one visit. For example, two areas may be treated together such as the crow's feet and frown lines, and 1-2 months later, treatment of forehead lines and an eyebrow lift may be performed.

Lower face. The lower face musculature performs essential functions of eating, drinking, and speaking. It is advisable to use caution when treating multiple muscles in the lower face concomitantly in one visit, as excessive weakening or unbalancing of muscles in this region can result in complications from functional impairment. When getting started in the lower face, a conservative approach to treatment of multiple muscles may be used, whereby only one muscle is treated at any given time and treatment areas are rotated every 3-4 months. For example, if upper lip lines and mental crease are of concern, the orbicularis oris m. may be treated initially, followed by treatment of the mentalis m. 3 months later, when the upper lip botulinum toxin effect has resolved. Once providers have gained experience with lower face treatments, they may elect to treat multiple lower face muscles in one visit, provided patients have no history of functional impairment from botulinum toxin treatment in any individual muscle previously treated. For example, the upper lip and chin may be treated concomitantly in one visit, and if there are no adverse effects, then the upper lip, chin, and DAO may be treated concomitantly at a subsequent visit.

Neck. There are multiple aesthetic indications for botulinum toxin treatment in the neck region such as anterior neck bands, posterior neck bands (Nefertiti Lift), and necklace lines. While the platysma m. does not perform essential functions in the neck, the muscles that lie deep to the platysma m. are responsible for functions such as neck stability and swallowing. When getting started with botulinum toxin treatments in the neck, it is advisable to treat only one neck indication in a given visit to reduce the risk of botulinum toxin affecting deeper muscles: either paired anterior bands, paired posterior bands, or necklace lines. Advanced injectors who have refined their injection technique and placement over time may consider treating multiple neck indications at one visit, taking care to limit the total dose for all indications in the neck to 40-50 units BTX or less.

 Tip

Botulinum toxin treatment of multiple muscles in the upper face concomitantly rarely has adverse effects. In the lower face, treatment of multiple muscles is approached more conservatively, adding areas incrementally over time to avoid functional impairment.

Other Common Applications

Providers using botulinum toxin for cosmetic applications may receive inquiries regarding specific injection techniques such as microtox and for treatment of other conditions such as headache and scars. In addition, certain cosmetic treatments may have therapeutic benefits such as improvement in depression. Some of these other common applications of botulinum toxin encountered in practice along with methods for treatment are discussed here.

Microtox

Microtox is a technique whereby multiple small wheals of dilute botulinum toxin are injected intradermally or subdermally. These low-dose injections relax muscle fibers of the superficial musculoapaneurotic system (SMAS) that attach to the underside of the dermis, reducing fine lines and improving skin texture, while preserving muscle function. For example, microtox in the midcheek can soften static cheek lines while leaving cheek risorius m. and buccinator m. functions unaffected. Additionally, microtox improves skin texture by reducing sebum production with atrophy of sebaceous and sweat glands and diminishes pore size. Microtox is commonly used in the forehead, neck, and cheeks.

Injections can be placed using standard botulinum toxin injection equipment or with autoinjectors that deliver microinjections using a stamping technique with multiple small gauge needles. One reported technique reconstitutes 100 units Botox with 2.5 mL saline, withdraws 0.5 mL solution in a 1 mL syringe (20 units), and mixes with 0.5 mL of lidocaine with epinephrine. Each 1 mL syringe is estimated to deliver 100 injections, and treatment of a region such as the neck typically requires 60 units Botox (3 syringes) staggered at 1-cm intervals. Some providers mix botulinum toxin together with hyaluronic acid in microtox treatments.

Depression

Botulinum toxin treatment of frown lines has been shown to improve depression in several clinical trials. Improved mood has been reported 6 weeks after treatment with botulinum toxin in the glabellar complex (30 units Botox in women and 40 units Botox in men) with results comparable effects of the antidepressant citalopram.

Antidepressant effects of botulinum toxin may be attributable to psychologic factors, whereby patients look better and feel better, or may be centrally mediated, where the balance of positive and negative neurochemical signaling is shifted. Magnetic resonance imaging has shown that botulinum toxin treatment of the glabellar complex inhibits neuronal signaling to brain areas involved in emotional processing. Decreased frowning from botulinum toxin in the glabellar complex may result in decreased negative emotional feedback to the brain. This is further supported by the finding that patients who did not even like the aesthetic effect of reduced frown lines from botulinum toxin treatment still experienced a lessening of their depression. Improvement in mood persisted for 6 months after cosmetic effects waned.

 Tip

Botulinum toxin treatment of the glabellar complex improves mood, in addition to aesthetic benefits of frown reduction and eyebrow elevation.

Scars

Botulinum toxin can reduce scar formation associated with surgical and traumatic wounds. Injections are placed around wounds (½ cm-2 cm from the wound margin, 8 units Botox per injection spaced 1 cm apart) within 24 hours of surgery. Relaxation of the surrounding musculature reduces tension on the wound, thereby minimizing scar formation. Commonly treated areas include the forehead, nose, chin, and glabella.

Botulinum toxin also improves cosmesis of mature scars. Intralesional botulinum toxin (5 units Botox per injection spaced 1 cm apart for a maximum of 15-50 units per scar, depending on the scar length) reduces the appearance of keloid and hypertrophic scars. A meta-analysis showed that intralesional botulinum toxin was more effective for the treatment of hypertrophic scars and keloids than intralesional corticosteroid and scar-related pain was reduced postinjection. Proposed mechanisms include suppressed fibroblast proliferation and reduced production of profibrotic factors by botulinum toxin.

Headache

For over a decade, botulinum toxin has been used as a preventative therapy for tension and migraine headaches and was FDA-approved in 2010 for chronic migraine prophylaxis. While relaxation of muscles contributes to reduced headache pain, botulinum toxin also reduces pain by inhibiting sensory neurons. Botulinum toxin inhibits release of pain mediators at sensory neurons, such as substance P and glutamate, in both the peripheral and central nervous system. Botulinum toxin has also proven useful in reducing postherpetic neuralgia pain, which is also mediated through this mechanism.

There are two approaches to headache prevention with botulinum toxin. The FDA-approved method, typically performed by neurologists and pain specialists, utilizes 155 units Botox broadly distributed in the upper face, temporalis, cervical paraspinal, occipital, and trapezius muscles. An alternative treatment approach entails targeting the facial areas associated with headache pain. Patients who present with focal pain in the glabellar complex and frontalis m. respond best with this method. Advantages of this technique include lower doses of botulinum toxin and nondisruption of stabilizing neck muscles.

Regardless of the treatment approach, care should be taken with patients whose headaches are easily triggered as treatment may precipitate a headache. Prophylactic use of a nonsteroidal anti-inflammatory medication immediately after treatment in patients easily triggered reduces the likelihood of injection-induced headache. Postponing treatment for patients presenting with acute headache at the time of treatment will help avoid exacerbation of symptoms. Subsequent treatments are performed at the early stages of recurrence of pain in 3½-4 months, the duration of cosmetic botulinum effects in the glabellar complex and frontalis muscles. Over time, the treatment interval can be refined such that botulinum toxin treatment is performed just prior to the recurrence of headaches, as determined by headache calendaring, which can render patients headache free.

Current Developments and New Products

DaxibotulinumtoxinA (DBTX)

DaxibotulinumtoxinA (Daxxify® manufactured by ReVance Therapeutics) has been FDA-approved for cosmetic use most recently. Like other botulinum toxins, daxibotulinumtoxinA consists of a core 150 kDa neurotoxin. It is formulated with polysorbate-20 and a peptide (RTP004) rather than human serum albumin, used in other botulinum toxin products for stabilization.

DaxibotulinumtoxinA has been FDA-approved to treat glabellar frown lines at a dose of 40 units. When administered in the glabella at a dose of 40 units, daxibotulinumtoxinA has a 6-month duration of action, similar to other toxins administered at higher than standard doses (see High-Dose Toxin chapter). Preliminary data also suggest that

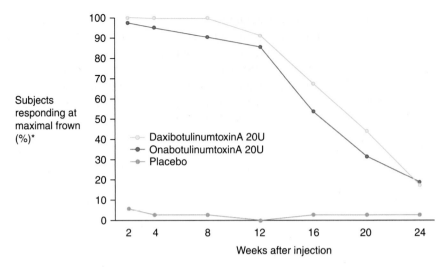

*Subjects responding is at least a 1-point improvement in Investigator Global Assessment—Facial Wrinkle Severity score

© Rebecca Small MD

FIGURE 8 ● Duration of botulinum toxin effect in the glabellar complex for frown line treatment using 20 units onabotulinumtoxinA vs 20 units daxibotulinumtoxinA. (Adapted from Carruthers J, et al. Injectable daxibotulinumtoxinA for the treatment of glabellar lines: a phase 2, randomized, dose-ranging, double-blind, multicenter comparison with onabotulinumtoxinA and placebo. *Dermatol Surg.* 2017;43(11):1321-1331. Figure 1. © 2017 American Society for Dermatologic Surgery.)

side effects of daxibotulinumtoxinA (40 units in the glabella) are similar to other botulinum toxins at standard doses but additional head-to-head and safety studies are needed.

When administered in the glabella at a dose of 20 units, daxibotulinumtoxinA has the same duration of action as 20 units of onabotulinumtoxinA (Botox). Figure 8 shows results from a head-to-head trial using 20 units onabotulinumtoxinA versus 20 units daxibotulinumtoxinA in which there were no statistical differences in clinical efficacy at any time point including weeks 4, 16, or 24. DaxibotulinumtoxinA appears to have a 1:1 dosing ratio with onabotulinumtoxinA and, as with other botulinum toxins, demonstrates an extended duration of action with escalating dose.

Combination Therapies

Facial aging is a multifactoral process involving many anatomic changes. In addition to hyperdynamic musculature contributing to formation of facial lines and wrinkles, facial contour changes as a result of volume loss and skin laxity, skin texture becomes rough, dyschromia and vascularities form, undesired hair growth occurs, and degenerative benign and malignant lesions form. Combining botulinum toxin with other minimally invasive procedures is often necessary to address these varied aspects of facial aging and achieve optimal aesthetic results. Furthermore, combining minimally invasive aesthetic treatments has synergistic effects, leading to rejuvenation that is superior to botulinum toxin or other therapies alone, often with longer duration of effects. For example, botulinum toxin is frequently combined with dermal fillers to restore structure and lift facial contours, and the combination procedure is called a "liquid lift." In addition to enhanced results, botulinum toxin also prolongs the duration of filler effects by reducing mechanical degradation in immobilized areas.

Therapies that can be safely combined with botulinum toxin are outlined in Table 4; grouped by regional treatments that are typically performed in the upper, middle, or lower facial regions, and full face treatments. Multiple treatments may be combined in a single visit or spaced sequentially over several visits based on provider skill and patient preference. In addition to enhancing outcomes and increasing the rapidity with which results are achieved, these types of multimodality visits also maximize provider time and increase office efficiency.

Providers must have a detailed understanding of facial anatomy, individual treatments, and interactions between treatments to safely and effectively combine minimally invasive therapies. The other books in the *Practical Guide* series serve to increase knowledge of these individual therapies (see Bibliography, Combining Aesthetic Treatments) and aesthetic training courses (eg, RSmdAestheticsTraining.com) bring these treatments together to help providers maximize outcomes in clinical practice.

Reimbursement and Financial Considerations

Cosmetic botulinum toxin treatments are not covered by insurance. Fees for botulinum toxin injections are either based on the number of units used or on the treatment area. Prices vary widely according to community norms in different geographic regions and range from $10-$25 per unit or $250-$600 per area. A fee structure based on pricing by treatment area has the advantage of focusing on outcomes rather than quantity of product used and allows compensation to be commensurate with skill level. For example, treatment of the levator labii superioris alaeque nasi m. for gummy smile is an advanced treatment area that typically requires 2 units BTX. Using a structure based on unit pricing, this may have a fee of $20, whereas it may have a fee of $250 based on treatment area pricing.

The Current Procedural Terminology (CPT) designations for botulinum toxin procedures are as follows:

Procedure	CPT Code
Chemodenervation of muscles innervated by the facial nerve	64612
Chemodenervation of neck muscles	64613
Chronic migraine paradigm	64615
Axillary primary hyperhidrosis	64650

Putting It All Together

There is a progression with learning botulinum toxin injection procedures akin to deconstruction and reconstruction of the face. Initially, facial movements are visually deconstructed into individual muscle actions and the focus is identification of target muscles only. For example, when treating the glabellar complex, the specific surface landmarks and location of the corrugator and procerus muscles are identified and muscle bulk assessed. Once providers can consistently identify individual muscles and their unique characteristics, the perspective then shifts. The face as a whole is assessed taking into account the functional relationships of multiple muscles, their synergy and antagonism, as well as facial symmetry. Using this holistic approach, aesthetic treatment plans can be created that globally soften and balance the effects of facial aging over time.

TABLE 4

Combination Minimally Invasive Aesthetic Procedures With Botulinum Toxin for Facial Rejuvenation

	Procedure	Indication	Mechanism and Examples	Combination Treatment Areas
Regional	**Dermal fillers**		Replacement of lost soft tissue volume: hyaluronic acid fillers are hydrophilic drawing water to plump tissues; biostimulant fillers increase synthesis of dermal matrix components such as collagen and elastin	
	Thinner	Fine lines	Volume restoration with hyaluronic acid products that have low G' (eg, Beloterro, Volbella, RHA 2)	Frown lines, mental crease, nasolabial folds, marionette lines
	Thicker	Lifting, augmentation and contouring	Volume restoration with hyaluronic acid and other products that have high G' (eg, Radiesse, Restylane-Lyft, Voluma)	Lifting eyebrows and jowls; augmenting chin; contouring malar and temporal hollows
	Threads		Dissolvable synthetic microfilament sutures such as polydioxanone (PDO), polylactic acid (PLA), and polycaprolactone (PCA)	
	Nonbarbed	Fine lines	Small caliber (eg, 30-27 gauge) smooth or twisted threads inserted into the dermis stimulate collagen production	Cheek and perioral lines
	Barbed	Lifting soft tissue	Large caliber (eg, 21-18 gauge) threads inserted into the subdermis lift tissue	Jowls, lax neck tissue, marionette lines and nasolabial folds
	Kybella	Focal adiposity	Lysis of adipose cells with synthetic deoxycholic acid (bile salt)	Submental and jowls
Full Face	**Resurfacing technologies**	Fine lines, rough skin texture, pigmentation	Wounding and removal of superficial skin layers in a controlled manner stimulate collagen production and dermal remodeling	

TABLE 4

Combination Minimally Invasive Aesthetic Procedures With Botulinum Toxin for Facial Rejuvenation *(Continued)*

	Procedure	Indication	Mechanism and Examples	Combination Treatment Areas
Full Face (Continued)	Microdermabrasion		Mechanical epidermal removal using abrasive element such as aluminum oxide crystals, diamond and abrasive tips	Face, neck, and chest
	Chemical peels		Chemical epidermal removal using acids such as glycolic acid, lactic acid, salicylic acid, Jessner's solution and trichloroacetic acid	Face, neck, and chest
	Microneedling		Microneedles (30 gauge) inserted 1-3 mm into the skin create small wounds that stimulate collagen production and dermal remodeling	Face, neck, and chest
	Ablative lasers		Vaporization of epidermis and superficial dermis using thermal energy (eg, erbium and carbon dioxide)	Face, neck, and chest
	Nonablative lasers and energy devices		Heating epidermis and dermis using thermal energy while leaving epidermis intact (eg, radiofrequency microneedling, fractional 1550 nm and Q-switched 1064 nm)	Face, neck, and chest
	Skin tightening technologies	Tightening, lifting, and contouring	Monopolar and bipolar radiofrequency use electrical current to heat the dermis creating zones of thermal coagulation and collagen contracture	Jowls and jawline contour
			Microfocused ultrasound heats the dermis creating zones of thermal coagulation and collagen contracture	Jowls and jawline contour

(Continued)

TABLE 4

Combination Minimally Invasive Aesthetic Procedures With Botulinum Toxin for Facial Rejuvenation *(Continued)*

	Procedure	Indication	Mechanism and Examples	Combination Treatment Areas
Full Face *(Continued)*	**Pigmentation and vascular technologies**	Solar lentigines, telangiectasias and erythema	Selective photothermolysis utilizes laser and light energy to heat and remove specific skin lesions such as IPL, vascular lasers (eg, 532 nm, 595 nm), and pigment lasers (eg, 755 nm, Q-switched 532 nm)	Face, neck, and chest
	Platelet-rich plasma (PRP)	Fine lines, skin texture and accelerates healing	Centrifugation of autologous blood separates out the platelet-rich fraction containing proteins, cytokines, and growth factors. Injection or topical application stimulates cell renewal and facilitate healing	Face, neck, and chest
	Topical products	Fine lines, skin texture and tone	Rejuvenation products such as sunscreen, retinoids, vitamin C, and growth factors protect against and treat ultraviolet-induced photodamage by stimulating cellular renewal and synthesis of dermal matrix components with regular application	Face, neck, and chest

G′ = Viscoelasticity, which is a physical property of dermal fillers. Dermal fillers with high G′ are firm, retain their shape and lift tissue.
IPL = Intense pulsed light

© Rebecca Small MD

The following chapters provide a structured approach to help providers acquire foundational knowledge and injection techniques for botulinum toxin treatment of individual muscles in preparation for hands-on injection. The intent of these chapters is to ensure providers can determine the exact location, depth, and dose for botulinum toxin injection of targeted muscles to optimize outcomes and minimize adverse effects by avoiding undesired muscles. The cases apply these principles to clinical practice and include common patient presenting complaints and demonstrate treatment in a variety of patients with different ethnicities, genders, ages, and facial characteristics.

The next step toward procedural proficiency, whether performing a new procedure or utilizing a new technique, requires observation of botulinum toxin injection followed by hands-on injection. Supervised injection by an experienced aesthetic clinician and ongoing mentorship for questions and management of adverse events is important and can be obtained through aesthetic training organizations.

Botulinum toxin procedures are one of the pillars of aesthetic practice, but success with facial aesthetics requires combining botulinum toxin with other minimally invasive procedures such as dermal fillers. High patient satisfaction with subtle natural results can be achieved when multiple modalities are integrated and each procedure adapted to the patient's unique anatomy. This patient-centered approach allows clinicians to achieve desired outcomes while further developing their aesthetic procedural expertise.

Treatment Areas

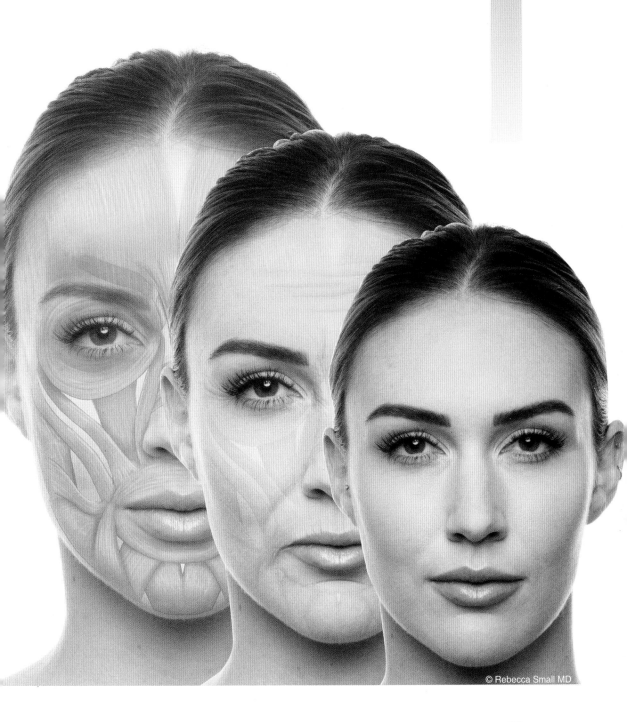

© Rebecca Small MD

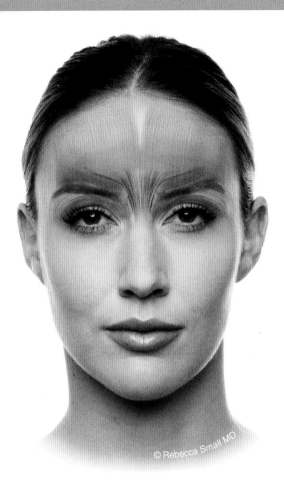

Chapter 1

© Rebecca Small MD

Key Points

Basic Treatment Area

Indications: Frown lines, Medial eyebrow elevation

Muscles Targeted: Glabellar complex

Frown Lines

Dynamic frown lines result from contraction of glabellar complex muscles. These lines convey irritation, frustration, or anger, and reduction of frown lines is one of the most common cosmetic complaints. Botulinum toxin treatment of the glabellar complex reduces frown lines and elevates the medial eyebrow by inhibiting contraction of these depressor muscles and smoothing the overlying skin.

Anatomy

- **Wrinkles.** Frown lines, or glabellar rhytids, are vertical lines between the medial eyebrows (Fig. 1-9A and see Anatomy section, Figs. 4, 5, and 8).
- **Muscles targeted**. Botulinum toxin frown line treatment targets the glabellar complex depressor muscles, which include the corrugator supercilii, procerus, depressor supercilii, and medial orbicularis oculi (see Anatomy section, Figs. 1 to 3). The corrugator and depressor supercilii muscles lie beneath the frontalis and procerus muscles (Fig. 1-1).
- **Muscle functions.** Contraction of the glabellar complex muscles draws the eyebrows medially and inferiorly. This muscle group is the major depressor of the upper face (see Anatomy section, Fig. 7).

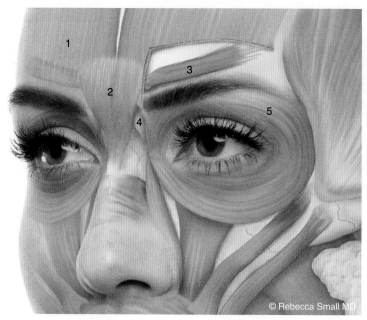

1. Frontalis m.   4. Depressor supercilii m.
2. Procerus m.   5. Orbicularis oculi m.
3. Corrugator supercilii m.

FIGURE 1-1 ● Glabellar complex detailed anatomy.
(© Rebecca Small MD.)

- **Muscles avoided.** The portion of the frontalis m. that is lateral to the corrugator muscles is avoided with treatment of the glabellar complex (Fig. 1-1). Upper eyelid levator muscles that attach on the supraorbital ridge of the lateral iris are also avoided.

Patient Assessment

- **General patient assessment** and **consultation** principles are outlined in the Introduction (see Introduction and Foundation Concepts section, Patient Selection and Aesthetic Consultation).
- **Dynamic** (with muscle contraction) and **static** (at rest) **frown lines** are assessed.
- **Concomitant muscle contraction in other facial areas** is assessed with frowning to determine if treatment of adjacent muscles is necessary such as the frontalis m. that forms horizontal forehead lines (Fig. 1-2), and nasalis m. that forms bunny lines (Fig. 1-3).

 Tip

Inform patients about adjacent muscle compensatory contraction to help achieve optimal reduction of frown lines and prevent hypertrophy of adjacent muscles.

Contraindications

- General injection-related and botulinum toxin-related contraindications are listed in the introduction (see Introduction and Foundation Concepts section, Contraindications).

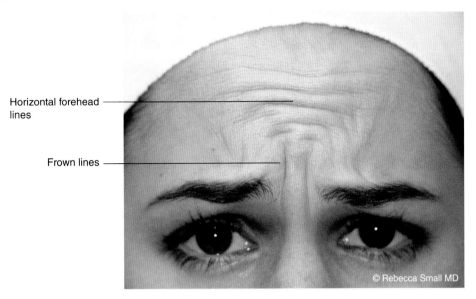

Horizontal forehead lines

Frown lines

FIGURE 1-2 ● Frontalis and glabellar complex muscle contraction with frowning. (© Rebecca Small MD.)

Eliciting Contraction of Muscles to Be Treated

Instruct the patient to perform any of the following expressions:
- "Frown like you are mad"
- "Concentrate"

Treatment Goals

- Complete inhibition of glabellar complex muscles.

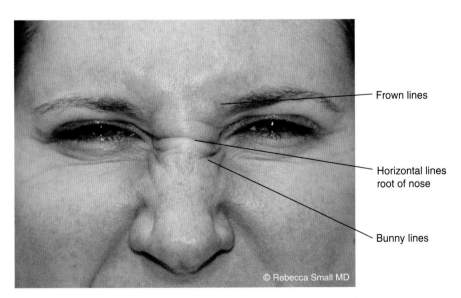

Frown lines

Horizontal lines root of nose

Bunny lines

FIGURE 1-3 ● Nasalis and glabellar complex muscle contraction with frowning. (© Rebecca Small MD.)

Reconstitution

- Botulinum toxin is abbreviated as BTX in this book and refers to onabotulinum-toxinA (Botox®), incobotulinumtoxinA (Xeomin®), and prabotulinumtoxinA (Jeuveau®). These products have similar 1:1 dosing ratios.
- Reconstitute 100 units of BTX powder with 4 mL of saline (see Introduction and Foundation Concepts section, Reconstitution Method).

Starting Doses

- Women: 20 units of BTX
- Men: 25 units of BTX

 Tip

Maximum combined botulinum toxin dose recommended for all treatments in a single session is 100 units BTX for providers just getting started, and may be greater than 100 units BTX per session for experienced providers.

Anesthesia

- Anesthesia is not necessary for most patients but an ice pack may be used if required.

Equipment for Treatment

- General botulinum toxin injection supplies (see Introduction and Foundation Concepts section, Equipment)
- Reconstituted botulinum toxin
- 30-gauge, 1-in needle

Procedure Overview

- Injections are placed within the frown line Safety Zone (Fig. 1-4). The Safety Zone is bounded laterally by vertical lines extending from the lateral irises to the hairline. Superiorly, it is bounded by a horizontal line approximately 2 cm above the supraorbital ridge, which typically corresponds to the lowest forehead wrinkle. The inferior

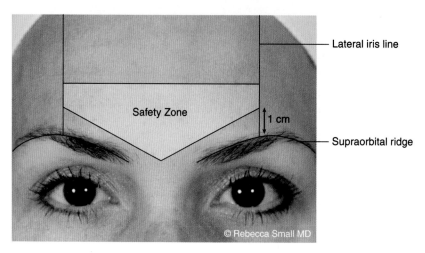

FIGURE 1-4 ● Frown line Safety Zone for botulinum toxin treatments. (© Rebecca Small MD.)

border of the Safety Zone extends from a point 1 cm below the glabellar prominence to a point 1 cm above the supraorbital ridge at the lateral iris line.
- An overview of injection sites and botulinum toxin doses for treatment of frown lines is shown in Figure 1-5.
- Botulinum toxin is injected intramuscularly for treatment of frown lines.

 Tip

Injecting inferior to the Safety Zone at the lateral iris line may affect eyelid levator muscles and increase the risk of blepharoptosis (droopy upper eyelid).

 Tip

Injecting lateral to the Safety Zone may affect the frontalis m. and increase the risk of eyebrow ptosis (droopy eyebrow).

Technique

1. Position the patient at a 60° angle.
2. Identify the frown line Safety Zone (Fig. 1-4).
3. Locate the glabellar complex muscles and identify the lateral margins of the corrugators that lie within the Safety Zone by instructing the patient to contract the muscles, using one of the facial expressions above.
4. Identify the injection sites (Fig. 1-5).
5. Ice for anesthesia (optional).
6. Prepare injection sites with alcohol and allow to dry.
7. The provider is positioned on the same side that is to be injected.
8. The lateral corrugator m. is injected while the glabellar complex muscles are contracted. Insert the needle 1-2 cm above the supraorbital ridge at the lateral margin of the corrugator m. within the Safety Zone. Angle the needle toward the procerus m. and insert to half the needle length (Fig. 1-6). Inject 2.5 units BTX with gentle, even plunger pressure as the needle is slowly withdrawn.

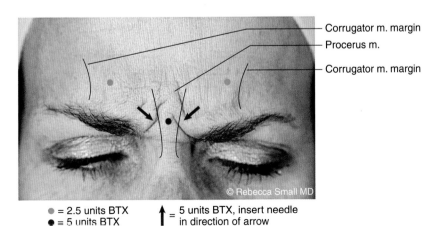

Corrugator m. margin
Procerus m.
Corrugator m. margin

● = 2.5 units BTX
● = 5 units BTX

↑ = 5 units BTX, insert needle in direction of arrow

FIGURE 1-5 ● Overview of botulinum toxin injection sites and doses for treatment of frown lines. (© Rebecca Small MD.)

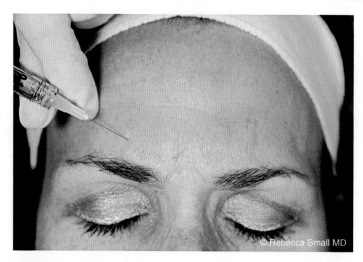

FIGURE 1-6 ● Lateral corrugator m. botulinum toxin injection technique. (© Rebecca Small MD.)

9. The medial corrugator m. injection is placed deep in the body of the corrugator m., approximately 1 cm medial and 1 cm inferior to the first injection site, closer to the eyebrow (Fig. 1-7). Angle the needle toward the procerus m. and insert to the hub. Inject 5 units BTX as the needle is slowly withdrawn.
10. Repeat the above injections for the contralateral side of the face.

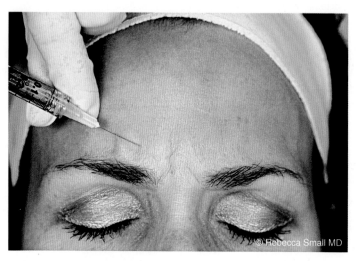

FIGURE 1-7 ● Medial corrugator m. botulinum toxin injection technique. (© Rebecca Small MD.)

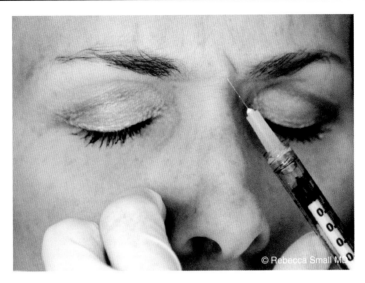

FIGURE 1-8 ● Procerus m. botulinum toxin injection technique. (© Rebecca Small MD.)

11. For the procerus m. injection, reposition to stand in front of the patient. While the glabellar complex muscles are contracted, approach inferiorly, direct the needle toward the glabella, insert to half the needle length, and inject 2.5-5 units BTX (Fig. 1-8).
12. Compress the injection sites firmly, directing pressure superiorly, away from the eye.

 Tip

Total number of botulinum toxin injection sites for treatment of the glabellar complex to reduce frown lines is typically 5.

Results

- **Reduction of dynamic frown lines** and **eyebrow elevation** are typically seen 3-5 days after botulinum toxin treatment, with maximal improvement at 2 weeks. Figure 1-9 shows contraction of the glabellar complex muscles before (Fig. 1-9A) and 1 month after (Fig. 1-9B) botulinum toxin injection. Botulinum toxin treatment of the glabellar complex results in 1-3 mm elevation of the eyebrows.

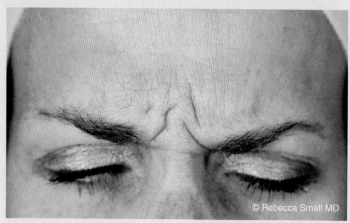

A. Before

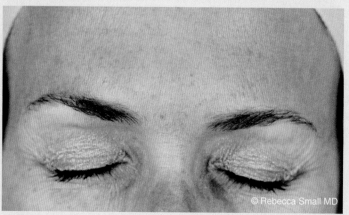

B. After

FIGURE 1-9 ● Frown lines before (**A**) and 1 month after (**B**) botulinum toxin treatment using 20 units BTX in the glabellar complex muscles, during maximal contraction. (© Rebecca Small MD.)

Duration of Effects and Treatment Intervals

- Muscle function in the treatment area gradually returns 3-4 months after botulinum toxin treatment.
- Subsequent frown line treatments with botulinum toxin may be performed when the glabellar complex muscles begin to contract, prior to lines returning to their pretreatment appearance.

Follow-ups and Management

Frown line reduction is assessed at a 2-week visit after botulinum toxin treatment. If frown lines persist, evaluate for the following common causes:

- **Glabellar muscle contraction.** Patients may have greater muscle mass than anticipated in the treatment area and additional botulinum toxin may be required to achieve desired results. Persistent muscle contraction can be corrected with a touch-up procedure using 5-10 units BTX, depending on the degree of glabellar m. activity present.

- **Broad glabellar complex musculature.** If the lateral margins of the corrugator muscles extend outside the Safety Zone lines, these portions of the corrugators will not receive treatment. The untreated portions of the corrugator muscles retain function and may cause medial frown lines. While fully immobilizing the entire corrugator will result in a more profound reduction of frown lines that is often sought by patients, it is advisable to avoid treating these active lateral portions of the corrugators when getting started with botulinum toxin injections because of the increased risks of blepharoptosis and eyebrow ptosis.

- **Frontalis muscle contraction with frowning.** In some patients, frontalis m. contraction contributes to frown line formation and botulinum toxin treatment of the frontalis m. may be required to achieve optimal frown line reduction.

- **Nasalis muscle contraction with frowning.** A horizontal line at the root of the nose may be visible, which is at the junction of the inferior procerus and nasalis muscles. Reducing this line usually requires treatment of both the glabellar complex and the nasalis muscles.

- **Static lines**. Superficial static lines that do not have an underlying depression typically show improvements after a few consecutive botulinum toxin treatments. Deep static lines that have an underlying depression visible at rest often require combination treatment with botulinum toxin and dermal fillers for demonstrable results (see Combining Aesthetic Treatments and Maximizing Results).

Eyebrow position and shape is also assessed at the 2-week follow-up visit. The whole eyebrow typically elevates with botulinum toxin treatment of the glabellar complex. Medial eyebrow elevation results from inhibition of the glabellar complex depressor function. Lateral eyebrow elevation results from compensatory contraction of the lateral frontalis in response to a small amount of botulinum toxin diffusion into the medial frontalis m. with glabellar complex treatment. While a moderate degree of lateral eyebrow elevation is desirable, excessive elevation may result in undesirable eyebrow shapes. Significant diffusion into the medial frontalis m. can occur with large doses of botulinum toxin in the glabellar complex muscles, or superior placement of toxin, resulting in the following undesirable eyebrow shapes:

- **"Peaked" or "quizzical" eyebrow shape.** The lateral frontalis m. can become hyperdynamic with excessive relaxation of the medial frontalis m. resulting in lateral pulling with a "peaked" unaesthetic shape to the eyebrows, and formation of crescent-shaped wrinkles above the lateral eyebrows. This is readily corrected with a touch-up dose in the lateral frontalis m. (see Horizontal Forehead Lines chapter).

Complications and Management

- General injection-related and botulinum toxin-related complications (see Introduction and Foundation Concepts section, Complications)
- Blepharoptosis (droopy eyelid)
- Eyebrow ptosis (droopy eyebrow)

Blepharoptosis, also referred to as eyelid droop, may occur with botulinum toxin treatment of the glabellar complex and is usually seen as a 2-3 mm lowering of the affected eyelid resulting in reduced eye aperture. It is almost always unilateral and most apparent at the end of the day with muscle fatigue. Figure 1-10 shows a patient 3 weeks after botulinum toxin treatment (at an outside facility) to glabellar complex muscles with a profound right-sided blepharoptosis and mild right eyebrow ptosis. Blepharoptosis is infrequent (1-5%) and temporary, typically resolving spontaneously within 6 weeks. While data on side-effects associated with high-dose toxin are limited, studies of 40 units DBTX suggest that, despite the longer duration of action, high-dose toxin may have the same incidence and duration of blepharoptosis as low dose toxin in the glabellar complex muscles.

It is important to distinguish eyelid ptosis from eyebrow ptosis, which can be done by assessing eye aperture. Eye aperture, also referred to as the palpebral fissure, is reduced with blepharoptosis and is unaffected with eyebrow ptosis.

Blepharoptosis results from migration of botulinum toxin through the orbital septum fascia to the levator palpebrae superioris m. of the upper eyelid. Some of the levator palpebrae superioris m. fibers pass up through the orbital septum and attach on the supraorbital ridge at the lateral iris. The risk of blepharoptosis is increased with botulinum toxin injection too close to the supraorbital ridge at the lateral iris line, as botulinum toxin may migrate into the levator palpebrae superioris m. at this point.

Blepharoptosis can be treated off-label using alpha-adrenergic eye drops such as naphazoline/pheniramine (eg, Naphcon-A) one drop four times per day in the affected eye, an over-the-counter medication typically used for season allergies, or with

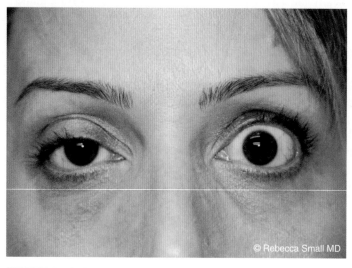

FIGURE 1-10 ● Right blepharoptosis. (© Rebecca Small MD.)

apraclonidine 0.5% solution (Iopidine) 1-2 drops three times per day, a prescription medication typically used for glaucoma. A newer prescription medication oxymetazoline 0.1% (Upneeq) one drop daily is the only on-label drug indicated for blepharoptosis (to be avoided with glaucoma). All of these medications cause contraction of the Müller m., a levator muscle of the upper eyelid, resulting in elevation of the upper eyelid. Side effects of these medications can include blurred vision and dry eyes.

Eyebrow ptosis can result from relaxation and descent of the frontalis muscle. The lower 2 cm of the frontalis m. primarily controls eyebrow height. Medial eyebrow ptosis can result from large botulinum toxin doses placed in the glabellar complex with diffusion into the medial frontalis m., from injecting superior to the Safety Zone, directly in the frontalis muscle. Other than ensuring the glabellar complex is fully treated, there is no correction for medial eyebrow ptosis and it self-resolves as botulinum toxin effects wear off. Lateral eyebrow ptosis can result from large botulinum toxin doses injected in the lateral frontalis m. and can be corrected with botulinum toxin injection in the superolateral orbicularis oculi m. to lift the lateral eyebrow (see Eyebrow Lift chapter).

Reducing the botulinum toxin dose for subsequent glabellar complex treatments and injecting within the Safety Zone can help prevent both of these complications.

Botulinum Toxin Treatment of Other Areas

Eyebrow position and height. Botulinum toxin treatments of the superolateral orbicularis oculi muscles (see Eyebrow Lift chapter) and the frontalis m. using the "V-shaped" injection pattern (see Horizontal Forehead Lines chapter) can further elevate the lateral eyebrow. This can be helpful for patients with dermatochalasis of the upper eyelids and patients desiring maximal lateral eyebrow elevation.

Horizontal forehead lines. Patients that form horizontal forehead lines when frowning usually require treatment of the frontalis m. in addition to the glabellar complex to smooth frown lines (see Horizontal Forehead Lines chapter).

Bunny lines. Patients that form bunny lines, particularly horizontal lines at the root of the nose (Fig. 1-3), when frowning require concomitant treatment of the nasalis m. and glabellar complex (see Bunny Line chapter). Bunny lines can become accentuated with botulinum toxin treatment of the glabellar complex over time due to compensatory nasalis m. contraction. In addition, lines of demarcation between treated glabellar muscles and an untreated nasalis m. can result in an unnatural "Botoxed" appearance rendering botulinum toxin treatments noticeable to others. For these reasons, concomitant bunny line and frown line treatments in patients who engage both muscle groups is recommended; ideally with every frown line treatment or every other treatment.

Combining Aesthetic Treatments and Maximizing Results

Deep static frown lines. Reduction of deep static frown lines that have an underlying depression usually requires combination treatment of botulinum toxin and dermal filler for correction. Figure 1-11 shows a patient with a deep static frown line before (Fig. 1-11A) and 1 month after (Fig. 1-11B) combination treatment with 20 units BTX in the glabellar complex and dermal filler treatment of the volume deficit.

RESULTS

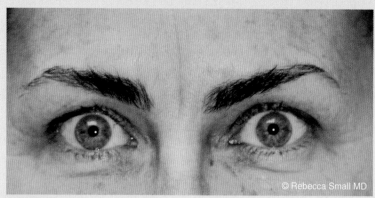

A. Before

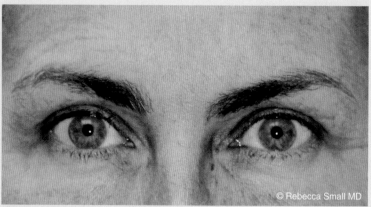

B. After

FIGURE 1-11 ● Deep static frown line before (**A**) and 1 month after (**B**) combination treatment with botulinum toxin using 20 units BTX in the glabellar complex muscles and dermal filler in the static frown line, at rest. (© Rebecca Small MD.)

Other Considerations

Depressed mood. Botulinum toxin treatment of frown lines has been shown to improve depressed mood (see Introduction and Foundation Concepts section, Depression). This effect may be attributable to psychologic factors or possibly to centrally mediated botulinum toxin effects.

Headache. Botulinum toxin is FDA-approved for prophylactic treatment of migraines and is also commonly used for tension headache prophylaxis (see Introduction and Foundation Concepts section, Headache). Patients with focal pain in the glabellar complex or frontalis m. respond well to relaxation of these muscles with botulinum toxin and results typically last for the duration of botulinum toxin effects, 3-4 months.

Pricing

Charges for botulinum toxin treatment of frown lines range from $200-$500 per treatment or $10-$25 per unit of BTX.

Case Studies

The techniques in this chapter for botulinum toxin treatment of the glabellar complex muscles are applied to patients with a variety of presentations encountered in clinical practice in the Cases section.

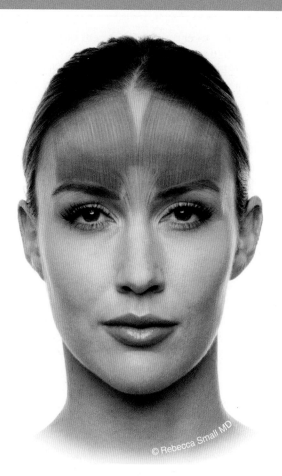

Chapter 2

Key Points

Intermediate Treatment Area

Indications: Horizontal forehead lines, Lateral eyebrow elevation

Muscles Targeted: Frontalis muscle

Contraindications: Eyebrow ptosis, Dermatochalasis of upper eyelid

Horizontal Forehead Lines

Dynamic horizontal forehead lines result from elevation of the eyebrows by contraction of the frontalis muscle. Botulinum toxin treatment of the frontalis m. reduces forehead lines by inhibiting muscle contraction and smoothing the overlying skin. In addition, certain injection techniques in the frontalis m. can produce lateral eyebrow elevation.

Anatomy

- **Wrinkles.** Horizontal forehead lines, or frontalis rhytids, course across the forehead (Fig. 2-7A and B, and see Anatomy section, Figs. 4, 5, and 8).
- **Eyebrow position and shape.** In women, high arched eyebrows located above the supraorbital ridge are usually desired. In men, a flat eyebrow shape is usually preferable, where the eyebrows lie on the supraorbital ridge (Figs. 2-7B and 2-8B, and see Eyebrow Lift chapter, Fig. 5-1A and B).

- **Muscles targeted.** Botulinum toxin horizontal forehead line treatment targets the broad frontalis m., which spans the forehead attaching laterally at the temporal fusion lines (see Anatomy section, Figs. 1 to 3). An aponeurosis (flat tendon) is located in the medial portion of the frontalis m. to a greater or lesser extent.
- **Muscle functions.** Frontalis m. fibers are oriented vertically, and contraction of this levator m. raises the eyebrows. The inferior 2 cm portion has the most significant effect on eyebrow height and shape (see Anatomy section, Fig. 7).

Patient Assessment

- **General patient assessment** and **consultation** principles are outlined in the Introduction (see Introduction and Foundation Concepts section, Patient Selection and Aesthetic Consultation).
- **Dynamic** (with muscle contraction) and **static** (at rest) **horizontal forehead lines** are assessed.
- **Dynamic** and **static eyebrow shape and height** are assessed.
- **Eyebrow ptosis** (low-set, droopy eyebrows) and **upper eyelid dermatochalasis** (skin laxity or redundancy) are assessed with the frontalis m. at rest. Figure 2-1 shows a patient with significant upper eyelid dermatochalasis. Patients with these conditions often have deep horizontal forehead lines as frontalis m. contraction is compensatory to elevate low set eyebrows and reduce upper eyelid skin laxity. While treatment with botulinum toxin will improve forehead lines, it can worsen eyebrow ptosis and eyelid dermatochalasis. When getting started with botulinum toxin injections, it is advisable to avoid treatment in patients with severe dermatochalasis and eyebrow ptosis. As experience is gained with injection placement and dosing in the frontalis m., providers may choose to treat patients with these more challenging presentations. Patients with low positioned eyebrows may tonically activate their frontalis m. unconsciously and their eyebrow position "at rest" may appear higher than it truly is. Instructing patients to close their eyes at the time of examination can help disengage the frontalis m. at rest allowing for assessment of eyebrow height with the frontalis m. fully relaxed.

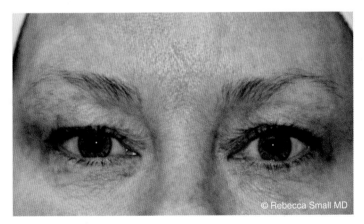

FIGURE 2-1 ● Dermatochalasis of the upper eyelid is a contraindication to horizontal forehead line treatment. (© Rebecca Small MD.)

- **Concomitant muscle contraction in other facial areas** is assessed with frontalis m. contraction. Treatment of the glabellar complex is necessary in almost every circumstance to ensure eyebrow height is maintained when treating the frontalis m. (see Frown Line chapter).
- **Eyebrow shape** is discussed before treating to determine botulinum toxin placement and help achieve patients' goals.

 Tip

Discuss opposing levator and depressor actions of muscles on the eyebrows at the time of consultation so patients understand the rationale behind treating adjacent muscle groups to preserve eyebrow height and achieve desired eyebrow shape.

Contraindications

- General contraindications to botulinum toxin treatments are listed in the Introduction (see Introduction and Foundation Concepts section, Contraindications).
- Specific contraindications to botulinum toxin treatment of forehead lines include: severe eyebrow ptosis and upper eyelid dermatochalasis.

Eliciting Contraction of Muscles to Be Treated

Instruct the patient to perform any of the following expressions:
- "Raise your eyebrows up like you are surprised"
- "Lift up your forehead"

Eliciting Relaxation of Muscles to Be Treated

- "Close your eyes, and slowly open without lifting up"

Treatment Goals

- Significant but not complete inhibition of the medial frontalis m. to reduce horizontal forehead lines with partial inhibition of the lateral frontalis m. to achieve a desirable eyebrow shape.

Reconstitution

- Botulinum toxin is abbreviated as BTX in this book and refers to onabotulinumtoxinA (Botox®), incobotulinumtoxinA (Xeomin®), and prabotulinumtoxinA (Jeuveau®). These products have similar 1:1 dosing ratios.
- Reconstitute 100 units of BTX powder with 4 mL of nonpreserved sterile saline (see Introduction and Foundation Concepts section, Reconstitution Method).

Starting Doses

- Women: 10-17.5 units BTX
- Men: 15-22.5 units BTX

 Tip

Maximum combined botulinum toxin dose recommended for all treatments in a single session is 100 units BTX for providers just getting started, and may be greater than 100 units BTX per session for experienced providers.

Anesthesia

- Anesthesia is not necessary for most patients but an ice pack may be used if required.

Equipment for Treatment

- General botulinum toxin injection supplies (see Introduction and Foundation Concepts section, Equipment)
- Reconstituted botulinum toxin
- 30-gauge, 0.5-in needle

Procedure Overview

- Place injections within the horizontal forehead line Safety Zone (Fig. 2-2). The Safety Zone is bounded by vertical lines at the lateral irises. The Safety Zone is bounded by a line 2 cm above the supraorbital ridge inferiorly, which typically lies along the lowest forehead wrinkle. A small area lateral to the vertical lines, approximately 2 cm inferior to the hairline, is also included in the Safety Zone. In men, or patients desiring a flat eyebrow shape, the small area lateral to the Safety Zone can be doubled in height, up to 4 cm below the hair line. Confining treatment to the Safety Zone minimizes the risk of eyebrow ptosis and preserves eyebrow shape and height.
- An overview of injection sites and botulinum toxin doses for treatment of horizontal forehead lines is shown in Figure 2-3 for a female patient and in Figure 2-4 for a male patient.
- The "V-shaped" injection pattern shown in Figure 2-3 minimizes botulinum toxin injection in the lateral portion of the frontalis m. and is typically used when treating women to elevate the lateral eyebrow and preserve the arched eyebrow shape. A flatter eyebrow shape can be achieved by injecting botulinum toxin more uniformly across the forehead and more inferiorly in the lateral frontalis muscle.
- Botulinum toxin placement and dosing lateral to the iris lines can be tricky. In general, it is better to have a result with peaked eyebrows (which can be corrected) than eyebrow ptosis.
- Botulinum toxin is injected intramuscularly for treatment of horizontal forehead lines.
- Avoid injecting too deeply and thus hitting the periosteum, which is painful and dulls the needle.

 Tip

Injecting inferior to the Safety Zone in the lateral frontalis m. and using high doses in the lateral frontalis m. increases the risk of lateral eyebrow ptosis.

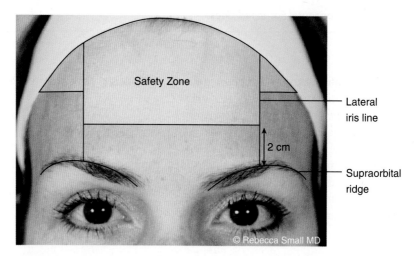

FIGURE 2-2 ● Horizontal forehead line Safety Zone for botulinum toxin treatments. (© Rebecca Small MD.)

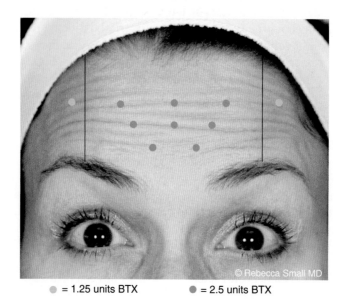

● = 1.25 units BTX   ● = 2.5 units BTX

FIGURE 2-3 ● Overview of BTX sites and doses for treatment of horizontal forehead lines in women. (© Rebecca Small MD.)

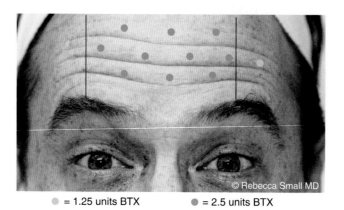

● = 1.25 units BTX   ● = 2.5 units BTX

FIGURE 2-4 ● Overview of botulinum toxin injection sites and doses for treatment of horizontal forehead lines in men. (© Rebecca Small MD.)

Technique

1. Position the patient at a 60° angle.
2. Identify the horizontal forehead line Safety Zone (Fig. 2-2).
3. Locate the frontalis m. and identify the ridges of the frontalis m. by instructing the patient to contract the muscle, using one of the facial expressions above.
4. Identify the injection sites (Fig. 2-3 or 2-4).
5. Ice for anesthesia (optional).
6. Prepare injection sites with alcohol and allow to dry.
7. The provider is positioned in front of the patient.
8. While the frontalis m. is contracted, insert the needle into the frontalis m. within the Safety Zone. The needle is angled at 30° to the forehead and the tip is inserted into the muscle ridge. Inject 2.5 units BTX with gentle, even plunger pressure (Fig. 2-5).
9. Continue laterally along each ridge of frontalis m. within the Safety Zone injecting 2.5 units BTX approximately 1 cm apart. Perform injections evenly across the forehead to achieve symmetry (Fig. 2-6).
10. The final injection is placed just lateral to the Safety Zone, within 2 cm of the hairline, at the maximal point of eyebrow elevation. Inject 1.25-2.5 units BTX based on the degree of contractility, and repeat for the contralateral side.
11. Compress the injection sites firmly, directing pressure superiorly away from the eye.

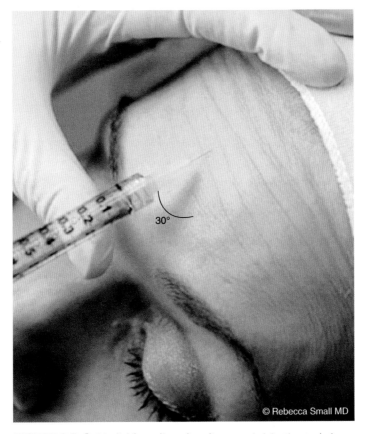

© Rebecca Small MD

FIGURE 2-5 ● Medial frontalis m. botulinum toxin injection technique. (© Rebecca Small MD.)

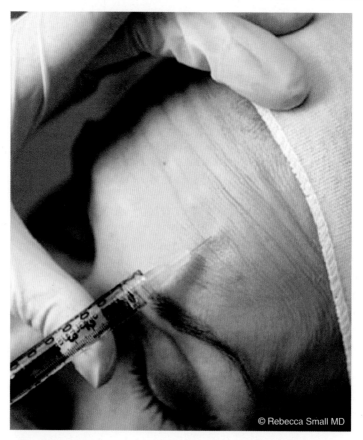

© Rebecca Small MD

FIGURE 2-6 ● Frontalis m. botulinum toxin injection technique. (© Rebecca Small MD.)

 Tip

Total number of botulinum toxin injection sites for treatment of the frontalis m. to reduce horizontal forehead lines is typically 10.

Results

- **Reduction of dynamic horizontal forehead lines** and **lateral eyebrow elevation** are typically seen 3-5 days after botulinum toxin treatment, with maximal improvement at 2 weeks. Figure 2-7 shows contraction of the frontalis m. before (Fig. 2-7A) and 1 month after (Fig. 2-7B) botulinum toxin injection in a woman desiring reduction of forehead wrinkles with preservation of arched brows. Figure 2-8 shows contraction of the frontalis m. before (Fig. 2-8A) and 1 month after (Fig. 2-8B) botulinum toxin injection in a man desiring reduction of forehead wrinkles with preservation of flat brows.

RESULTS

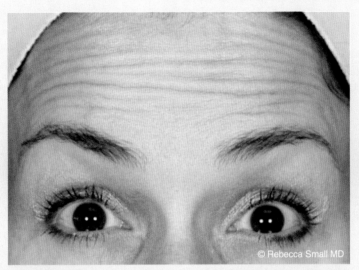

A. Before

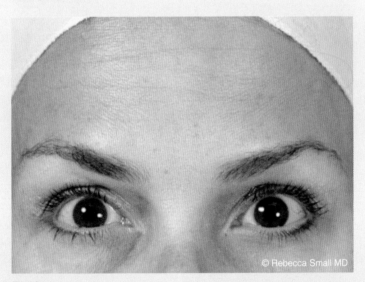

B. After

FIGURE 2-7 ● Horizontal forehead lines before **(A)** and 1 month after **(B)** botulinum toxin treatment using 22.5 units BTX in the frontalis m., during maximal contraction. (© Rebecca Small MD.)

RESULTS

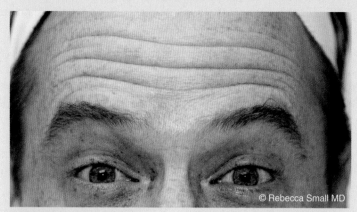

A. Before

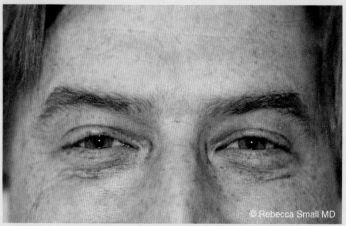

B. After

FIGURE 2-8 ● Horizontal forehead lines before **(A)** and 1 month after **(B)** botulinum toxin treatment using 22.5 units BTX in the frontalis m., during maximal contraction. (© Rebecca Small MD.)

Duration of Effects and Treatment Intervals

- Muscle function in the treatment area gradually returns 3-4 months after treatment.
- Subsequent horizontal forehead line treatments with botulinum toxin may be performed when the frontalis m. begins to contract before the lines return to their pretreatment appearance.

Follow-ups and Management

Forehead lines, eyebrow symmetry, shape, and height at rest and with active eyebrow elevation are assessed at a 2-week visit after botulinum toxin treatment. The following patient concerns may be encountered at that visit:

Persistent horizontal forehead lines. If forehead lines are present, assess for the following:

- **Dynamic lines.** Patients may have greater muscle mass than anticipated in the treatment area and additional botulinum toxin may be required to achieve desired results. Persistent muscle contraction can be corrected with a touch-up procedure using 5-7.5 units BTX, depending on the degree of frontalis m. activity present.
- **Static lines.** While static lines typically show improvements after several consecutive botulinum toxin treatments, combination treatment can achieve more rapid results (see Combining Aesthetic Treatments and Maximizing Results).

Peaked eyebrow shape, "Quizzical brow", or "Spock brow". Peaked eyebrows are most noticeable with animation and are due to excessive contraction of the lateral frontalis muscle. This can occur in patients with inherently strong lateral frontalis muscles, if lateral frontalis m. botulinum toxin injections were omitted, injections were placed too superiorly near the hair line, or if the botulinum toxin doses used in the lateral frontalis m. were too small and ineffective. Peaked eyebrows can be corrected with 1.25-2.5 units BTX placed just inferior to the lateral Safety Zone, in line with the

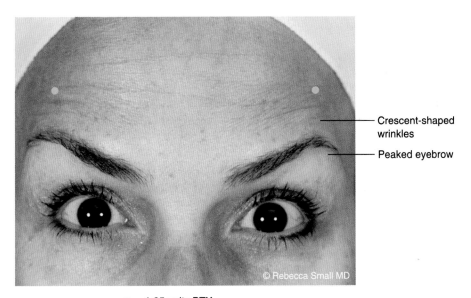

Crescent-shaped wrinkles

Peaked eyebrow

● = 1.25 units BTX

FIGURE 2-9 ● Peaked eyebrows and crescent-shaped wrinkles corrected with botulinum toxin. (© Rebecca Small MD.)

most peaked portion of the eyebrow. Figure 2-9 shows a patient actively contracting the frontalis m. demonstrating peaked eyebrows bilaterally 2 weeks after treatment with 22.5 units BTX in the frontalis m.; and associated injection sites for correction. Figure 2-7B shows the same patient 2 weeks after receiving 1.25 units BTX above each peaked eyebrow (4 weeks after the initial treatment) and represents the final result.

New wrinkles. Patients may report new crescent-shaped wrinkles above the lateral eyebrow, or new wrinkles at the hairline, with botulinum toxin treatment of the frontalis muscle. Initially, these are dynamic but may become static over time. The desired compensatory contraction of the lateral frontalis m. that results in lateral eyebrow elevation can also result in the formation of lateral eyebrow wrinkles. Figure 2-9 demonstrates crescent-shaped wrinkles above the lateral eyebrow. These wrinkles can be softened with a botulinum toxin touch-up procedure in the lateral frontalis muscle; the same procedure used for peaked eyebrows.

> **Tip**
>
> Dynamic horizontal forehead lines commonly seen at the hairline and above the lateral brow, as well as peaked-eyebrow shape, may require a touch-up procedure at the 2-week visit.

Complications and Management

- General injection-related and botulinum toxin-related complications (see Introduction and Foundation Concepts section, Complications)
- Eyebrow ptosis (droopy eyebrow)
- Eyebrow asymmetry
- Blepharoptosis (droopy upper eyelid)

Eyebrow ptosis is one of the most significant complications from botulinum toxin treatment of the frontalis muscle. Excessive botulinum toxin doses in the frontalis m. or placement inferiorly in the lateral frontalis m. can result in eyebrow ptosis. Patients often present with a complaint of heaviness of the upper eyelid on the affected side. Eyebrow ptosis may be unilateral or bilateral and is typically seen as a lowering and flattening of the affected eyebrow, while the palpebral fissures remain unaffected and symmetric (unlike blepharoptosis, where the palpebral fissure on the affected side is reduced). The medial, lateral, or entire eyebrow may be affected, depending on the region of frontalis m. that is involved. Figure 2-10 shows a patient before (Fig. 2-10A) and 2 weeks after (Fig. 2-10B) botulinum toxin treatment with 20 units BTX in the frontalis m. demonstrating medial eyebrow ptosis and flattening of the eyebrow. Eyebrow ptosis resolves spontaneously as botulinum toxin effects wear off. Medial eyebrow ptosis may be improved by treating the glabellar complex with botulinum toxin if this area is untreated (see Frown Lines chapter). Lateral eyebrow ptosis may be improved by treating the superolateral orbicularis oculi m. with botulinum toxin and lifting the lateral eyebrow (see Eyebrow Lift chapter).

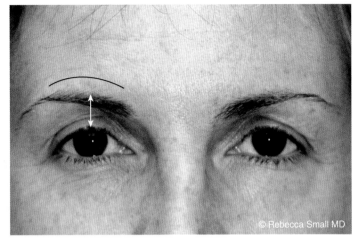

A

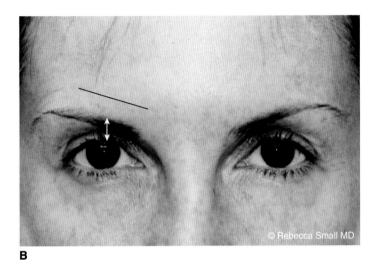

B

FIGURE 2-10 ● Eyebrow position before **(A)** and 2 weeks after **(B)** botulinum toxin treatment using 20 units BTX in the frontalis m. demonstrating eyebrow ptosis and flattening, at rest. (© Rebecca Small MD.)

Eyebrow asymmetry may result from eyebrow ptosis and/or a peaked eyebrow. Figure 2-11 shows a patient with eyebrow asymmetry 2 weeks after botulinum toxin treatment using 22.5 units BTX in the frontalis muscle. The patient has a lower, flatter right eyebrow and a peaked left eyebrow. This asymmetry may be corrected by treating the superolateral orbicularis oculi m. on the right side with botulinum toxin to lift the lateral eyebrow (see Eyebrow Lift chapter) and treating the lateral frontalis on the patient's left side to reduce the peaked eyebrow.

Blepharoptosis is uncommon with frontalis m. treatments. It can result from inferior placement of botulinum toxin at the lateral iris line with diffusion into the levator muscles of the upper eyelid. See Frown Lines chapter for additional information on blepharoptosis and management strategies.

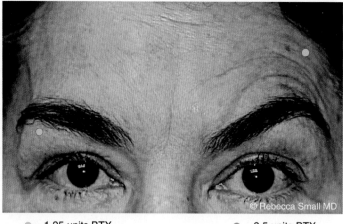

● = 1.25 units BTX   ● = 2.5 units BTX

FIGURE 2-11 ● Eyebrow asymmetry and correction with botulinum toxin. (© Rebecca Small MD.)

Botulinum Toxin Treatment of Other Areas

Eyebrow position and height. Balancing depressor and levator m. effects on the eyebrows with botulinum toxin treatments optimizes eyebrow position and height. Reduced frontalis m. levator function can be balanced by botulinum toxin treatment of the opposing eyebrow depressor muscles, such as the glabellar complex (see Frown Lines chapter), lateral orbicularis oculi (see Crow's Feet chapter), and superolateral orbicularis oculi (see Eyebrow Lift chapter) muscles, thereby reducing the risk of eyebrow ptosis. The specific muscle groups treated will depend on the patient's desired eyebrow height and shape.

 Tip

The frontalis m. is almost always treated concommittantly with the glabellar complex, and in some cases with the superolateral orbicularis oculi muscles as well, to balance depressor and levator m. functions.

Combining Aesthetic Treatments and Maximizing Results

Superficial static horizontal forehead lines. Combining botulinum toxin treatments with resurfacing procedures such as fractional ablative lasers or chemical peels reduces superficial static lines.

Deep static horizontal forehead lines. When an underlying horizontal forehead line depression is present, combination treatment with dermal fillers helps achieve more dramatic results (see *A Practical Guide to Dermal Filler Procedures*). Fillers are particularly useful for treatment of crescent-shaped forehead lines located above the lateral eyebrow as these cannot be readily corrected with botulinum toxin alone due to the risk of eyebrow ptosis.

Other Considerations

Headache. Botulinum toxin is FDA-approved for prophylactic treatment of migraines and is commonly used for tension headaches as well (see Introduction and Foundation Concepts section, Headache). Patients with focal pain in the glabellar complex or frontalis m. region usually respond well to relaxation of these muscles with botulinum toxin and results typically last 3-4 months.

Scars. Botulinum toxin has been used as an adjuvant treatment to improve cosmesis of surgical and traumatic wounds on the forehead. Botulinum toxin injections placed around wound sites minimize movement and tension on wound margins, facilitating reapproximation and healing (see Introduction and Foundation Concepts section, Scars).

Pricing

Charges for botulinum toxin treatment of horizontal forehead lines range from $200-$500 per treatment or $10-$25 per unit of BTX.

Case Studies

The techniques in this chapter for botulinum toxin treatment of the frontalis m. are applied to patients with a variety of presentations encountered in clinical practice in the Cases section.

Chapter 3

Key Points

Core Treatment Area

Indications: Crow's feet, Lateral eyebrow lift

Muscles Targeted: Orbicularis oculi muscle (lateral)

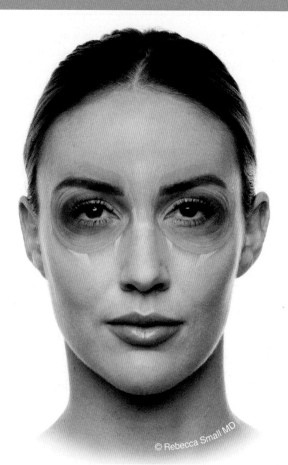

Crow's Feet

Dynamic crow's feet result from contraction of the lateral orbicularis oculi m. with smiling, laughing, and squinting. Botulinum toxin treatment of the lateral orbicularis oculi m. reduces crow's feet and elevates the lateral eyebrow by inhibiting contraction of this depressor m. and smoothing the overlying skin.

Anatomy

- **Wrinkles.** Crow's feet, or lateral canthal rhytids, radiate laterally from the eye (Fig. 3-7A and see Anatomy section, Figs. 4, 5, and 8).
- **Muscles targeted.** Botulinum toxin crow's feet treatment targets the lateral orbital portion of the orbicularis oculi muscle. The orbicularis oculi m. is a superficial, thin, sphincteric muscle that encircles the eye (see Anatomy section, Figs. 1 to 3). It has a palpebral portion covering the eye and an orbital portion around the eye (see Lower Eyelid Wrinkles chapter, Fig. 4-2).

- **Muscle functions.** Different regions of the orbicularis oculi m. have different functions and contribute to formation of different periocular wrinkles (see Anatomy section, Fig. 7). The lateral orbital portion of the orbicularis oculi m. functions as lateral eyebrow depressor, forms crow's feet, and is responsible for forceful eye closure. The superolateral orbital portion also functions as a lateral eyebrow depressor and forms infrabrow lines (see Eyebrow Lift chapter). The palpebral portion of the orbicularis oculi m. functions to gently close the eyelids both voluntarily and involuntarily as part of the blink reflex and forms lower eyelid wrinkles (see Lower Eyelid Wrinkles chapter). The deep lacrimal portion of the orbicularis oculi m. contributes to lacrimal function.
- **Muscles avoided.** The zygomaticus major and minor muscles, which are lip and cheek levators, are avoided with treatment of crow's feet. These muscles lie deep to the orbicularis oculi m. and are most closely approximated to the orbicularis oculi m. at the zygomatic arch (see Anatomy section, Figs. 1 to 3).

Patient Assessment

- **General patient assessment** and **consultation** principles are outlined in the Introduction (see Introduction and Foundation Concepts section, Patient Selection and Aesthetic Consultation).
- **Blepharoplasty** and other facial surgery history are reviewed. Periocular surgery may alter muscle attachments increasing the risk of complications such as lip ptosis from unintended botulinum toxin effect in lip levator muscles. Ophthalmologic history is obtained, including keratorefractive (LASIK) surgery, as this may increase the risk of dry eyes.
- **Dynamic** (with muscle contraction) and **static** (at rest) crow's feet are assessed.
- **Concomitant muscle contraction in other facial areas** is assessed with smiling to determine if botulinum toxin treatment of adjacent areas is necessary including: infrabrow lines due to superolateral orbicularis oculi m., lower eyelid wrinkles due to inferior orbicularis oculi m., and bunny lines due to nasalis m. contraction (Fig. 3-1).

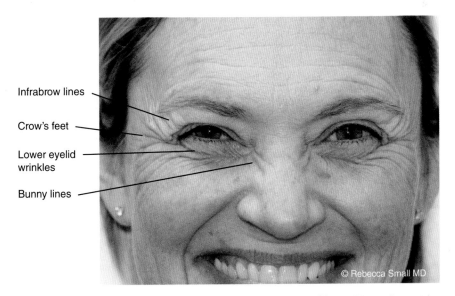

Infrabrow lines

Crow's feet

Lower eyelid wrinkles

Bunny lines

FIGURE 3-1 ● Formation of infrabrow lines, lower eyelid wrinkles and bunny lines with smiling. (© Rebecca Small MD.)

Tip

Evaluate and discuss contraction of adjacent muscles at the time of consultation so patients understand the rational behind treating these muscles to prevent formation of lines in adjacent areas over time.

Contraindications

- General injection-related and botulinum toxin-related contraindications are listed in the introduction (see Introduction and Foundation Concepts section, Contraindications).

Eliciting Contraction of Muscles to Be Treated

Instruct the patient to perform any of the following expressions:
- "Cheesy grin" or "big smile"
- "Squint like the sun is in your eyes"
- "Wink"

Treatment Goals

- Nearly complete inhibition of the lateral orbicularis oculi muscle.

Reconstitution

- Botulinum toxin is abbreviated as BTX in this book and refers to onabotulinumtoxinA (Botox®), incobotulinumtoxinA (Xeomin®), and prabotulinumtoxinA (Jeuveau®). These products have similar 1:1 dosing ratios.
- Reconstitute 100 units of BTX powder with 4 mL of nonpreserved sterile saline (see Introduction and Foundation Concepts section, Reconstitution Method).

Starting Doses

- Women: total (bilateral) dose is 15-20 units BTX
- Men: total (bilateral) dose is 20-25 units BTX

 Tip

Maximum combined botulinum toxin dose recommended for treatment of all areas in a single session is 100 units BTX for providers just getting started, and may be greater than 100 units BTX per session for experienced providers.

Anesthesia

- Anesthesia with ice is not recommended as it vasoconstricts and can obscure blood vessels.

Equipment for Treatment

- General botulinum toxin injection supplies (see Introduction and Foundation Concepts section, Equipment)
- Reconstituted botulinum toxin
- 30- or 32-gauge, 0.5-in needle

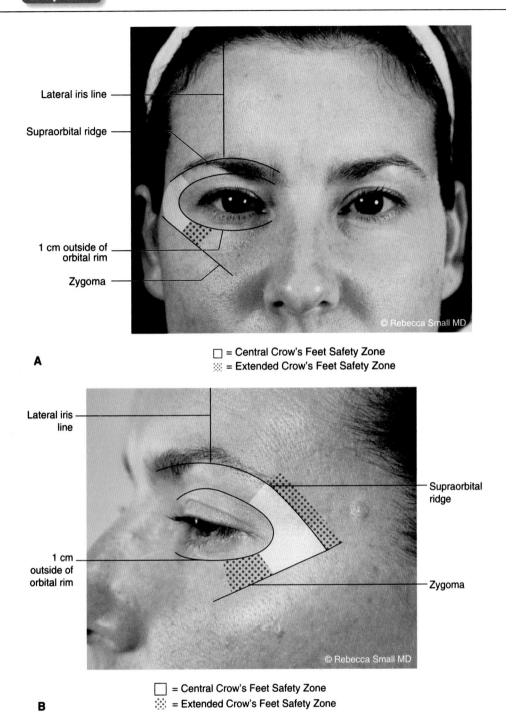

A   □ = Central Crow's Feet Safety Zone
    ▒ = Extended Crow's Feet Safety Zone

B   □ = Central Crow's Feet Safety Zone
    ▒ = Extended Crow's Feet Safety Zone

FIGURE 3-2 ● Crow's feet Safety Zone for botulinum toxin treatments: front (**A**) and lateral (**B**) views. (© Rebecca Small MD.)

Procedure Overview

- Place injections within the crow's feet Safety Zone (Fig. 3-2A and B). The Safety Zone is 1 cm outside the orbital rim, above the level of the superior margin of the zygoma, and extends under the eyebrow to the lateral iris line. Botulinum toxin is concentrated within the central crow's feet Safety Zone, but injections may also be placed in the extended Safety Zone according to patients' anatomy.

- An overview of injection sites and botulinum toxin doses for treatment of crow's feet is shown in Figure 3-3. Injection sites are located in the "ridges" or "hills" of contracted muscle.
- Patterns of crow's feet vary, some extend superiorly toward the eyebrow and others extend inferiorly toward the cheek. Optimal treatment of the crow's feet is achieved by adapting the injection technique to the patient's specific crow's feet pattern.
- Botulinum toxin is injected subdermally for treatment of crow's feet. It is important to place injections superficially in this region as the orbicularis oculi m. overlies other muscles, which, if affected by botulinum toxin, can result in lip and cheek ptosis, and smile asymmetry. Subdermal injection can be achieved using the following technique: instruct the patient to contract the muscle in the treatment area by smiling and insert the needle just below the skin. Once the needle tip is inserted, instruct the patient to relax the muscle by slowly releasing their smile and inject botulinum toxin to raise a visible wheal.
- The lateral canthal region has many veins and bruising is common. Veins are best seen and avoided using oblique lighting. If numerous vessels are visible in the treatment area, ecchymosis may be reduced by injecting a series of continuous wheals, where each injection is placed at the border of the previous wheal. If bruising occurs, apply firm pressure and ice for a few minutes during the procedure.

 Tip

Injecting medial to the crow's feet Safety Zone near the orbital rim at the lateral canthus can increase the risk of diplopia due to deep migration of botulinum toxin in the extraocular muscles.

 Tip

Injecting inferior to the crow's feet Safety Zone below the superior margin of the zygoma, injecting deeply, or using high doses, increase the risk of cheek and lip ptosis and smile asymmetry.

Technique

1. Position the patient at a 60° angle.
2. Identify the crow's feet Safety Zone and palpate the orbital rim (Fig. 3-2).
3. Locate the orbicularis oculi m. by instructing the patient to contract the muscles using one of the facial expressions above.
4. Identify the injection sites (Fig. 3-3).
5. Prepare injection sites with alcohol and allow to dry.
6. The provider is positioned on the side that is to be injected.
7. While the lateral orbicularis oculi m. is contracted, insert the needle into the orbicularis oculi muscle ridge within the Safety Zone, near the lateral canthal line (Fig. 3-4). Inject 2.5 units BTX subdermally with gentle plunger pressure, using the technique described in the Procedure Overview.
8. The second injection site is approximately 5 mm superior to the first injection site. Inject 2.5 units BTX (Fig. 3-5).

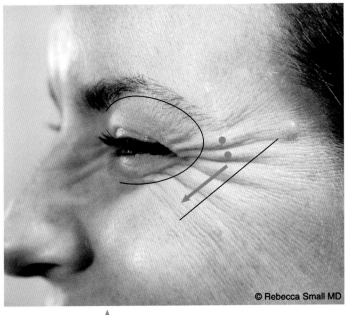

● = 2.5 units BTX   ↑ = 2.5 units BTX, insert needle in direction of arrow

FIGURE 3-3 ● Overview of botulinum toxin injection sites and doses for treatment of crow's feet. (© Rebecca Small MD.)

9. The third injection site is approximately 5 mm inferior to the first injection site. The needle is angled inferiorly and threaded superficially to the hub. Inject 2.5 units BTX as the needle is withdrawn (see Fig. 3-6).
10. Repeat injections for the contralateral orbicularis oculi muscle.
11. Compress the injection sites firmly, directing pressure away from the eye.

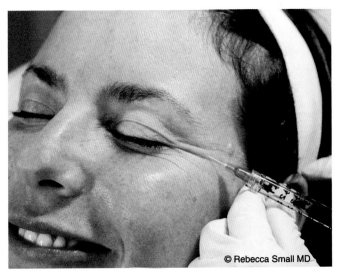

FIGURE 3-4 ● First lateral orbicularis oculi m. botulinum toxin injection. (© Rebecca Small MD.)

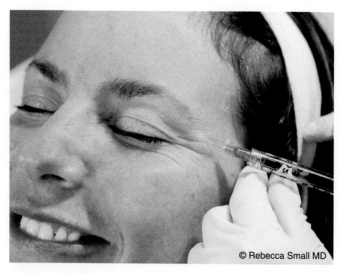

© Rebecca Small MD

FIGURE 3-5 ● Second lateral orbicularis oculi m. botulinum toxin injection. (© Rebecca Small MD.)

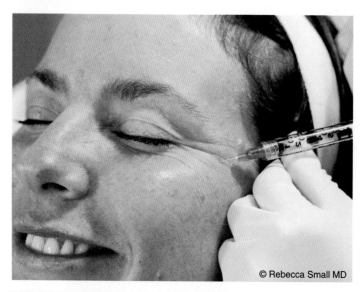

© Rebecca Small MD

FIGURE 3-6 ● Third lateral orbicularis oculi m. botulinum toxin injection. (© Rebecca Small MD.)

 Tip

Total number of botulinum toxin injection sites for treatment of the lateral orbicularis oculi m. to reduce crow's feet is typically 6.

Results

- **Reduction of crow's feet** and **lateral eyebrow elevation** are typically seen 3-5 days after botulinum toxin treatment, with maximal improvement at 2 weeks. Figure 3-7 shows contraction of the lateral orbicularis oculi before (Fig. 3-7A) and 1 month after (Fig. 3-7B) botulinum toxin injection.

RESULTS

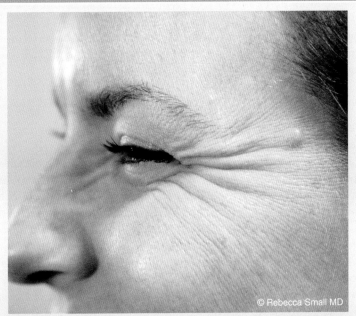

A. Before

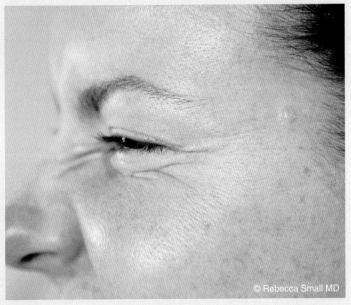

B. After

FIGURE 3-7 ● Crow's feet before **(A)** and 1 month after **(B)** botulinum toxin treatment using 15 units BTX in the lateral orbicularis oculi muscles, during maximal contraction. (© Rebecca Small MD.)

Duration of Effects and Treatment Intervals

- Muscle function in the treatment area gradually returns 2½-3 months after botulinum toxin treatment.
- Subsequent crow's feet treatments with botulinum toxin may be performed when the orbicularis oculi m. begins to contract, before the lines return to their pretreatment appearance.

Follow-ups and Management

Crow's feet reduction is assessed at a 2-week visit after botulinum toxin treatment. If crow's feet persist, evaluate for the following common causes:

- **Orbicularis oculi muscle contraction.** Patients may have greater muscle mass than anticipated in the treatment area and additional botulinum toxin may be required to achieve desired results. Persistent muscle contraction can be corrected with a touch-up procedure using 2.5-10 units BTX, depending on the degree of orbicularis oculi m. activity present. Reassess the treatment area 2 weeks after the touch-up procedure.
- **Cheek muscle contraction.** Some patients will retain a few wrinkles inferior to the crow's feet treatment area, which are most noticeable with smiling (see Fig. 3-7B). These wrinkles are due to appropriately retained function of the zygomatic muscles and require no additional treatment.
- **Static lines.** If static crow's feet are present, patients may require several consecutive botulinum toxin treatments for results to be seen. Combining botulinum toxin with other minimally invasive aesthetic procedures can offer enhanced results for treatment of static crow's feet (see Combining Aesthetic Treatments and Maximizing Results).

Wrinkles in adjacent areas can result from compensatory muscle contraction in adjacent untreated muscles. Common areas to evaluate include the following:

- **Bunny lines** resulting from contraction of the nasalis m. can be treated with botulinum toxin (see Bunny Lines chapter).
- **Lines under the eyebrow** can result from contraction of the superolateral orbicularis oculi muscle. Botulinum toxin may be placed in the superolateral orbicularis oculi m. to reduce these wrinkles (see Eyebrow Lift chapter).
- **Lower eyelid wrinkles** can result from contraction of the medial preseptal orbicularis oculi m., and a stepwise approach can be used to reduce these wrinkles:
  - Decreasing the botulinum toxin dose in the third injection site at subsequent visits can reduce lower eyelid wrinkles resulting from medial orbicularis oculi contraction.
  - If this does not effect enough reduction in lower eyelid wrinkles, botulinum toxin may be placed directly in the preseptal orbicularis oculi muscle (see Lower Eyelid Wrinkles chapter).

Complications and Management

- General injection-related and botulinum toxin-related complications (see Introduction and Foundation Concepts section, Complications)
- Bruising
- Photophobia
- Periorbital flattening

- Lip and cheek ptosis with resultant smile asymmetry
- Oral incompetence with resultant drooling and impaired speaking, eating, and drinking
- Impaired blink reflex
- Ectropion of the lower eyelid (eyelid margin eversion)
- Lagophthalmos (incomplete eyelid closure)
- Xerophthalmia (dry eyes)
- Corneal damage
- Diplopia (double vision)
- Strabismus (crossed eyes)
- Globe trauma

Bruising (ecchymosis) is the most common complication seen with treatment of crow's feet due to numerous superficial periocular veins. Bruises can range in size from pinpoint needle insertion marks to quarter-sized bruises or hematomas, and if extravasated blood spreads, a "black eye" seen as a large infraocular ecchymotic crescent may occur. The time for resolution of a bruise depends on the patients' physiology and the size of the bruise. Larger bruises can be visible for 2 weeks. Strategies for bruise prevention are listed in the Introduction and Foundation Concepts section, Preprocedure Checklist. Immediate application of ice and pressure to a bruise can minimize bruising. Vascular lasers such as 532 nm, 595 nm pulsed dye, and intense pulsed light devices can accelerate bruise resolution significantly.

Photophobia is uncommon and when it occurs is usually mild. It typically results from reduced squinting strength. Using sun protective measures such as sunglasses and hats can alleviate this problem.

Periorbital flattening with full effacement of all crow's feet may occur if the lateral orbicularis m. is excessively weakened with large botulinum toxin doses. A distinct line demarcating the superior margin of the zygomaticus muscles against the flaccid lateral orbicularis oculi m. may be seen with smiling creating an unaesthetic appearance. This will self-resolve as botulinum toxin effects wear off, but dermal filler treatment in the zygoma can increase volume and restore a natural contour in this area.

Lip and cheek ptosis causing smile asymmetry can occur with injections placed deeply and inferiorly below the superior margin of the zygoma and with large doses weakening the upper lip levator muscles. The zygomaticus major m. is most frequently involved, which is closely approximated to the orbicularis oculi m. at the zygomatic arch. Botulinum toxin effect in the zygomaticus major m. typically presents with lip and cheek ptosis, similar to Bell's palsy, without oral incompetence. Patients who have undergone facial plastic surgery may be at increased risk of zygomaticus m. involvement because of altered anatomy. While severe complications of **oral incompetence** due to lip levator relaxation may also occur with resultant drooling and impaired speaking, eating, or drinking, they are extremely rare. Placement of botulinum toxin superficially and above the margin of the zygoma reduces the risk of these complications.

Impaired eyelid function and altered lower eyelid position, such as ectropion and lagophthalmos, are very rare and can occur with high botulinum toxin doses that excessively weaken the palpebral orbicularis oculi m., or if botulinum toxin is placed too close to the eyelid. **Xerophthalmia,** which is extremely rare, can result from impaired eyelid function with reduced lacrimal flow, or may be secondary to ectropion and lagophthalmos. Patients who have had LASIK surgery may be more susceptible to xerophthalmia. **Corneal damage** such as keratitis sicca (corneal desiccation) and punctate keratitis (corneal ulcerations) can result from prolonged dry eyes and corneal exposure. **Diplopia** and **strabismus** can occur with deep migration of botulinum toxin into extraocular muscles. **Globe trauma** is a risk with injections placed near the eye. There are no corrective treatments for most ocular complications; however, they will spontaneously resolve as botulinum toxin effects diminish. Consultation with an ophthalmologist is advisable with ocular complications.

Botulinum Toxin Treatment of Other Areas

When several muscle groups simultaneously engage during a particular facial expression, treatment of one muscle with the exclusion of the other muscles can result in compensatory contraction of the untreated muscles. Over time, this can result in formation or worsening of lines in the untreated areas. Patients who form lines in the following areas when smiling usually require concomitant treatment with the lateral orbicularis oculi m. to prevent worsening of lines in these other areas due to compensatory contraction:

- **Lower eyelid wrinkles** from preseptal orbicularis oculi m. contraction (see Lower Eyelid Wrinkles chapter)
- **Infrabrow lines** from superolateral orbicularis oculi m. contraction (see Eyebrow Lift chapter)
- **Bunny lines** from nasalis m. contraction (see Bunny Line chapter)

Combining Aesthetic Treatments and Maximizing Results

Static crow's feet. Botulinum toxin in the orbicularis oculi m. can be combined with the following minimally invasive aesthetic procedures to reduce static crow's feet:

- Dermal fillers can be used to restore volume in the zygoma area or in discrete crow's feet. Figure 3-8 shows a patient with static crow's feet, before (Fig. 3-8A) and after (Fig. 3-8B) combination treatment with botulinum toxin in the lateral orbicularis oculi m. and dermal filler treatment of the zygoma.
- Resurfacing procedures such as fractional ablative lasers or chemical peels are helpful adjunctive treatments for superficial static lines. Figure 3-9 shows a patient with superficial static crow's feet before (Fig. 3-9A) and after (Fig. 3-9B) combination treatment with botulinum toxin in the lateral orbicularis oculi m. and periocular fractional ablative laser resurfacing.
- Topical products such as retinoids (eg, tretinoin), growth factors, and alpha hydroxy acids (eg, glycolic and lactic acid) have been shown to reduce fine lines when used consistently over a period of months. While prescription strength retinoids are effective, they can be associated with a retinoid dermatitis. Less active retinoids such as over-the-counter retinol are more commonly used in the periocular area.

RESULTS

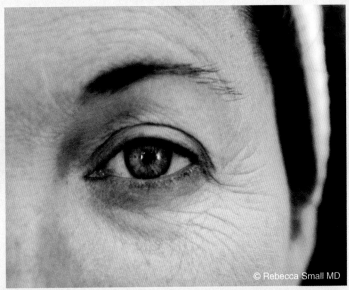

A. Before

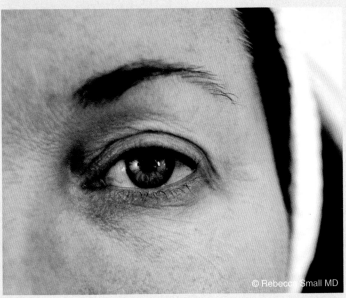

B. After

FIGURE 3-8 ● Static crow's feet before **(A)** and after **(B)** combination treatment with botulinum toxin using 15 units BTX in the orbicularis oculi m. and dermal filler in the zygoma, at rest. (© Rebecca Small MD.)

RESULTS

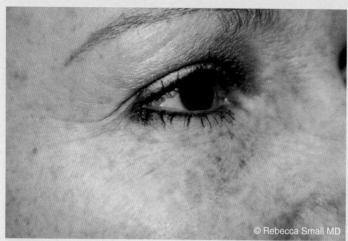

A. Before

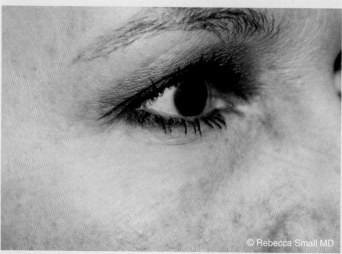

B. After

FIGURE 3-9 ● Static crow's feet before **(A)** and after **(B)** combination treatment with botulinum toxin using 15 units BTX in the orbicularis oculi m. and periocular fractional ablative laser resurfacing, at rest. (© Rebecca Small MD.)

Pricing

Charges for botulinum toxin treatment of crow's feet range from $200-$500 per treatment or $10-$25 per unit of BTX.

Case Studies

The techniques in this chapter for botulinum toxin treatment of the orbicularis oculi m. are applied to patients with a variety of presentations encountered in clinical practice in the Cases section.

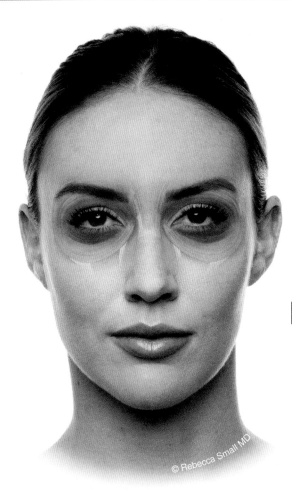

© Rebecca Small MD

Chapter 4

Key Points

Advanced Treatment Area

Indications: Lower eyelid wrinkles, Palpebral aperture enlargement and rounding of the eye shape, Lower eyelid muscle bulge

Muscles Targeted: Orbicularis oculi muscle (palpebral)

Contraindications: Dermatochalasis of lower eyelid, Abnormal snap test, Lower eyelid edema, Infraorbital festoons, Lagophthalmos, Scleral show, Ectropion

Lower Eyelid Wrinkles

Contraction of the inferior portion of the orbicularis oculi m. contributes to formation of lower eyelid wrinkles, typically seen with smiling, laughing, and squinting. Treatment of the inferior orbicularis oculi m. with botulinum toxin focally inhibits contraction, which results in reduction of lower eyelid wrinkles, opening of the eye aperture, and if present, reduces lower eyelid muscle bulge.

Anatomy

- **Wrinkles.** Lower eyelid wrinkles, or infraocular rhytids, course horizontally under the lower eyelid (Figs. 4-1B and 4-11A). They are often associated with a lower eyelid muscle bulge seen with animation, referred to as a "jelly roll" (Fig. 4-1A). Lower eyelid wrinkles may be accentuated by botulinum toxin treatment of crow's feet.
- **Muscles targeted.** The orbicularis oculi m. has an orbital portion, which surrounds the eye, and a palpebral portion, which covers the eye. The palpebral portion is further divided into the preseptal fibers and the pretarsal fibers that form the eyelids (Fig. 4-2). Lower eyelid wrinkle treatments with botulinum toxin target the inferior preseptal region of the palpebral orbicularis oculi muscle. Jelly roll treatments target the inferior pretarsal region of the palpebral orbicularis oculi muscle.

93

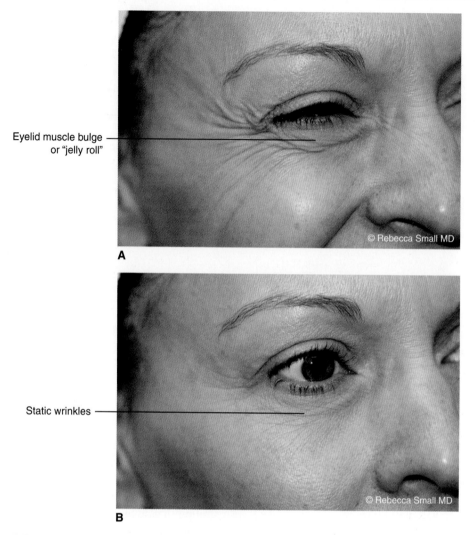

Eyelid muscle bulge or "jelly roll"

A

Static wrinkles

B

FIGURE 4-1 ● Lower eyelid dynamic wrinkles with muscle bulge ("jelly roll") **(A)** and static wrinkles **(B)**. (© Rebecca Small MD.)

- **Muscle functions.** Different regions of the orbicularis oculi m. have different functions and contribute to formation of different periocular wrinkles (see Crow's Feet and Eyebrow Lift chapters). The palpebral portion of the orbicularis oculi m. functions to gently close the eyelids both voluntarily and involuntarily as part of the blink reflex, facilitates drainage of lymphatic fluid, and forms lower eyelid wrinkles. The pretarsal region of the palpebral orbicularis m. forms the lower eyelid muscle bulge or jelly roll.

Patient Assessment

- **General patient assessment** and **consultation** principles are outlined in the Introduction (see Introduction and Foundation Concepts section, Patient Selection and Aesthetic Consultation).
- **Facial surgery** and skin resurfacing procedural history is obtained. It is advisable to **use caution** in patients who have had previous lower eyelid surgery (eg, blepharoplasty) or aggressive lower eyelid resurfacing (eg, ablative laser resurfacing or deep

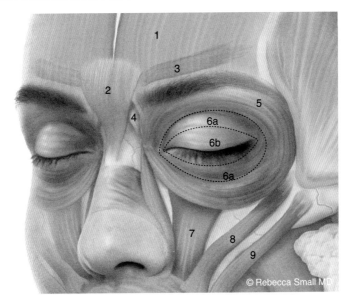

1. Frontalis m.
2. Procerus m.
3. Corrugator supercilii m.
4. Depressor supercilii m
5. Orbicularis oculi m.
    (orbital portion)

6. Orbicularis oculi m. (palpebral
portion)
  a. Preseptal
  b. Pretarsal
7. Levator labii superioris m.

FIGURE 4-2 ● Periocular detailed anatomy. (© Rebecca Small MD.)

chemical peels) as they may exhibit lagophthalmos, excessive lower eyelid scleral
show, or an ectropion, which contraindicate treatment with botulinum toxin. Ophthalmologic history including keratorefractive surgery (LASIK) is obtained as these
patients may have a greater risk of dry eyes.

- **Lower eyelid edema** history is obtained. Patients who report lower eyelid edema or
  "puffiness" at baseline will likely experience worsening edema with botulinum toxin
  treatment of the lower eye lids and are not candidates for treatment.
- **Dynamic** (with muscle contraction) assessments of the lower eyelid are made including the following:
  - **Lower eyelid wrinkles** are evaluated while the patient contracts the lower eyelid
    muscles (Fig. 4-1A). Botulinum toxin injection techniques described in this chap-
    ter focus on treatment of lower eyelid wrinkles at, or lateral to, the midpupillary
    line not medial to the midpupillary line.
  - **Lower eyelid muscle bulge or "jelly roll"** is also assessed while the patient con-
    tracts the lower eyelid muscles (Fig. 4-1A). Botulinum toxin injection of the lower
    eyelid can soften this muscle bulge and increase the palpebral aperture, which can
    widen and round the eye shape. It's important to note that in certain Asian cultures,
    the lower eyelid muscle bulge is a hallmark of beauty, referred to as the "charming
    roll," and determining patient preferences at the time of consultation, as with all
    aesthetic treatments, is essential when developing a treatment plan.
- **Static** (at rest) assessments of the lower eyelid are made including the following:
  - **Lower eyelid wrinkles** are assessed with the face at rest (Fig. 4-1B). Static lower
    eyelid wrinkles not associated with laxity respond well to botulinum toxin treatment.
  - **Palpebral aperture** (ie, the distance between upper and lower eyelid margins)
    and **eyeshape** are assessed at rest. If desired, botulinum toxin injection in the
    lower eyelid can increase eye aperture and round the eye shape.

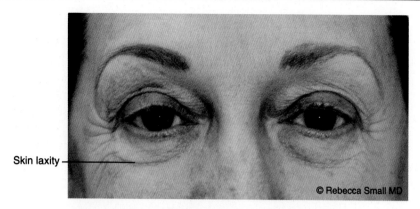

Skin laxity

© Rebecca Small MD

FIGURE 4-3 ● Laxity (dermatochalasis) of the lower eyelid is a contraindication to botulinum toxin treatment of the lower eyelid. (© Rebecca Small MD.)

- **Lower eyelid dermatochalasis,** or skin laxity is clinically evident as loose folds of the skin and wrinkles in the lower eyelid area (Fig. 4-3). Botulinum toxin treatment of the lower eyelid may exacerbate dermatochalasis and treatment should be avoided in patients with obvious skin laxity. Surgery is often required to improve lower eyelid wrinkles due to severe skin laxity.
- **Elasticity of the lower eyelids** is assessed using the **snap test.** It is performed by grasping the skin of the lower eyelid between the thumb and the first finger, pulling the skin gently away from the eye and releasing (Fig. 4-4). If the skin recoils in less than 3 seconds, the snap test is normal and botulinum toxin treatment may be performed. If the skin recoils slowly (more than 3 seconds), the lower eyelid has insufficient elasticity and should not be treated with botulinum toxin.
- **Infraorbital festoons,** or lower eye bags, are soft tissue bulges that are visible at rest (Fig. 4-5). The orbital septum, a facial layer that helps to retain infraorbital fat pads, weakens with age. Eye bags are typically due to bulging of the infraorbital fat pad as a result of a weakened orbital septum. The orbicularis oculi m. also supports the inferior orbital septum and weakening of this muscle with botulinum toxin can exacerbate festooning. Treatment with botulinum toxin should be avoided in patients with eye bags.

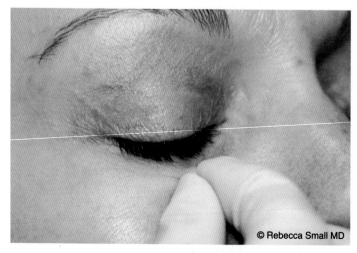

© Rebecca Small MD

FIGURE 4-4 ● Snap test for evaluation of lower eyelid elasticity. (© Rebecca Small MD.)

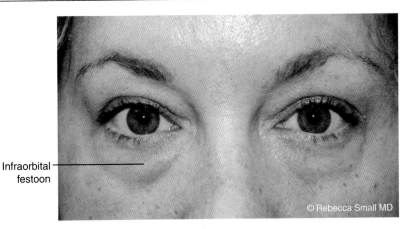

Infraorbital
festoon

FIGURE 4-5 ● Infraorbital festoons are a contraindication to botulinum toxin treatment of the lower eyelids. (© Rebecca Small MD.)

- **Scleral show** refers to the crescent of white sclera visible between the iris and the lower eyelid margin at rest with forward level gaze. Scleral show is due to lower lid retraction and, while a small amount of scleral show is common and a normal finding with forward gaze, excessive sclera show of more than 2 mm is a contraindication to botulinum toxin treatment of the lower eyelid.
- **Ectropion**, which is eversion of lower eyelid margin, is a contraindication for botulinum toxin treatment of the lower eyelid.
- **Lagophthalmos** is incomplete closure of eyelids. This can be assessed by instructing the patient to "roll their eyes upward" while trying to keep their eyelids closed. Figure 4-6 shows a patient with a history of a blepharoplasty demonstrating lagophthalmos with upward gaze. This is a contraindication to botulinum toxin treatment of the lower eyelids.
- **Concomitant formation of lower eyelid wrinkles with muscle contraction in other facial areas** is assessed. Patients that form lower eyelid wrinkles with nasalis m. (see Bunny Lines chapter) or orbicularis oculi m. contraction (see Crow's Feet chapter) show greater reduction in lower eyelid wrinkles when these muscles are concomitantly treated with the inferior palpebral orbicularis oculi muscle.

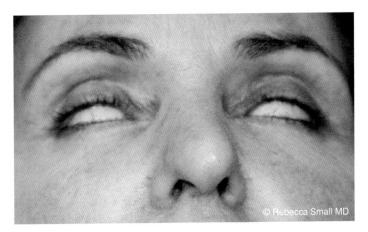

FIGURE 4-6 ● Incomplete eyelid closure (lagophthalmos), shown in a patient with a history of a blepharoplasty, is a contraindication to botulinum toxin treatment of the lower eyelids. (© Rebecca Small MD.)

Contraindications

- General contraindications to botulinum toxin treatments are listed in the Introduction (see Introduction and Foundation Concepts section, Contraindications).
- Specific contraindications to botulinum toxin treatment of lower eyelid wrinkles include: dermatochalasis of the lower eyelid, abnormal snap test, lower eyelid edema, infraorbital festoons, lagophthalmos, scleral show, and ectropion.

Eliciting Contraction of Muscles to Be Treated

Instruct the patient to perform any of the following expressions:
- "Cheesy grin" or "Big smile"
- "Squint like the sun is in your eyes"

Treatment Goal

- Partial inhibition of the inferior palpebral orbicularis oculi muscle.

Reconstitution

- Botulinum toxin in this book is abbreviated as BTX and refers to onabotulinumtoxinA (Botox®), incobotulinumtoxinA (Xeomin®), and prabotulinumtoxinA (Jeuveau®). These products have similar 1:1 dosing ratios.
- Reconstitute 100 units of BTX powder with 4 mL of nonpreserved sterile saline (see Introduction and Foundation Concepts section, Reconstitution Method).

Starting Doses

- Women and men: total (bilateral) dose is 2.5 units BTX

 Tip

Maximum combined botulinum toxin dose recommended for all treatments in a single session is 100 units BTX for providers just getting started, and may be greater than 100 units BTX per session for experienced providers.

Anesthesia

- Anesthesia with ice is not recommended because it vasoconstricts and can obscure blood vessels.

Equipment for Treatment

- General botulinum toxin injection supplies (see Introduction and Foundation Concepts section, Equipment)
- Reconstituted botulinum toxin
- 30- or 32-gauge 0.5-in needle

Procedure Overview

- An overview of injection sites and botulinum toxin doses for treatment of lower eyelid wrinkles is shown in Figure 4-7. Two injections are usually performed for each eye, one medial (Fig. 4-7A) and one lateral (Fig. 4-7B).
- The lateral injection site has a greater risk of lowerlid retraction and ectropion due to botulinum toxin weakening of the pretarsal orbicularius oculi muscle. Providers getting started with botulinum toxin injections may choose to start with injection of the medial site only, to reduce the risk of complications.

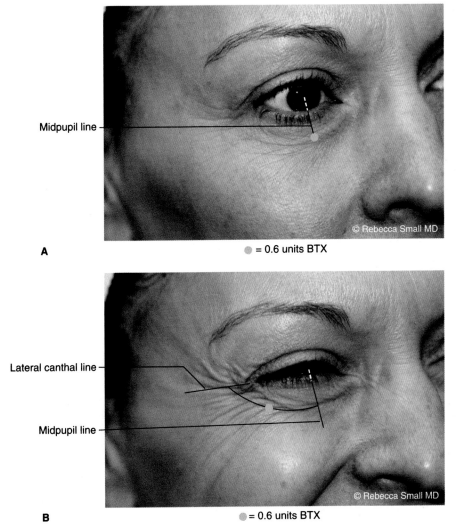

Midpupil line

A   ◉ = 0.6 units BTX

Lateral canthal line

Midpupil line

B   ◉ = 0.6 units BTX

FIGURE 4-7 ● Overview of botulinum toxin injection sites and doses for treatment of lower eyelid wrinkles. The medial injection is placed with the muscles at rest **(A)** and the lateral injection is placed during orbicularis oculi m. contraction **(B)**. (© Rebecca Small MD.)

- Botulinum toxin is injected subdermally for treatment of lower eyelid wrinkles. These injections require a light touch as the orbicularis oculi m. is a superficial muscle and the lower eyelid skin is very thin.
- For patients with long eyelashes that obscure the medial injection site, instruct them to "roll their eyes upward" while keeping their eyelids closed to visualize the injection site.
- The inferior eyelid region has many tiny veins that are best seen and avoided using oblique lighting.

 Tip

Injecting too superiorly, less than 3 mm from the lower eyelash margin, may increase the risk lower eyelid ectropion and lagophthalmos due to excessive weakening of the palpebral obicularis oculi muscle.

Tip

It is advisable to stabilize during injections by placing the nondominant hand against the patient's head to reduce the risk of globe trauma from unexpected patient movement.

Technique

1. Position the patient at a 60° angle.
2. Identify the lateral canthal and midpupillary lines (Fig. 4-7B). Palpate the orbital rim (Fig. 4-8).
3. Prepare injection sites with alcohol and allow them to dry.
4. The provider is positioned on the side that is to be injected.
5. **Medial lower eyelid injection.** The medial lower eyelid injection is located in the midpupillary line. Either lower eyelid wrinkles or the jelly roll may be treated, not both in the same visit.
   - Lower eyelid wrinkles are treated using an injection point 5 mm inferior to the eyelid margin in the preseptal orbicularis oculi muscle (Fig. 4-7A). While the muscles are at rest and patient's eyes are closed, angle the needle medially, almost parallel to the skin, and insert the needle tip subdermally just under the skin. Inject 0.6 units BTX to raise a wheal (Fig. 4-9).
   - Jelly roll is treated closer to the lower lid margin using the same method, at an injection point 3 mm inferior to the eyelid margin in the pretarsal orbicularis oculi muscle.
6. **Lateral lower eyelid injection.** The lateral lower eyelid injection site is located midway between the first injection site and the lateral canthal line.
   - Lower eyelid wrinkles are treated using an injection point 1 cm inferior to the eyelid margin (Fig. 4-7B). While the orbicularis oculi m. is contracted, angle the needle towards the nasal ala, almost parallel to the skin, and insert the needle tip subdermally just under the skin. Inject 0.6 units BTX to raise a wheal (Fig. 4-10).
   - Jelly roll treatment does not require a lateral lower eyelid injection.

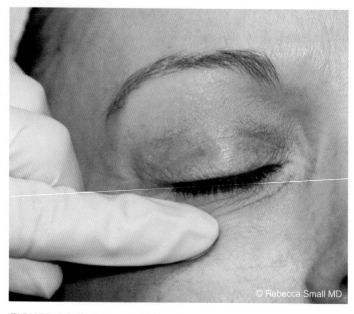

FIGURE 4-8 ● Palpation of the infraorbital rim. (© Rebecca Small MD.)

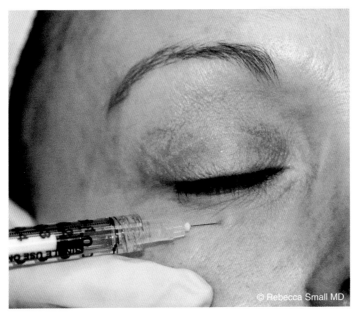

FIGURE 4-9 ● Medial botulinum toxin injection of the inferior orbicularis oculi muscle. (© Rebecca Small MD.)

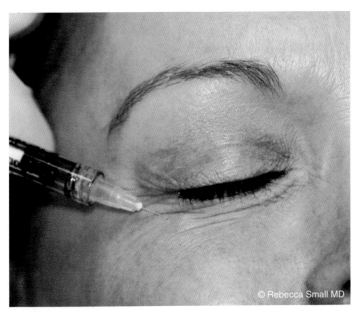

FIGURE 4-10 ● Lateral botulinum toxin injection of the inferior orbicularis oculi muscle. (© Rebecca Small MD.)

7. Repeat injections for the contralateral inferior orbicularis oculi muscle.
8. Compress the injection sites, directing pressure away from the eye.

 Tip

Total number of botulinum toxin injection sites for treatment of the palpebral orbicularis oculi m. to reduce lower eyelid wrinkles or lower eyelid muscle bulge is typically 4.

Results

- **Reduction of lower eyelid wrinkles**, "jelly roll," and **eye aperture enlargement** are typically seen 3-5 days after botulinum toxin treatment, with maximal improvements at 2 weeks. Figure 4-11 shows static lower eyelid wrinkles before (Fig. 4-11A) and 1 month after (Fig. 4-11B) botulinum toxin injection. Unlike botulinum toxin treatments in other regions of the face, both static and dynamic lower eyelid wrinkles usually respond well to treatment.

Duration of Effects and Treatment Intervals

- Muscle function in the treatment area gradually returns 2.5-3 months after botulinum toxin treatment.
- Subsequent lower eyelid treatments with botulinum toxin may be performed when the orbicularis oculi m. begins to contract, before lines and wrinkles return to their pretreatment appearance.

RESULTS

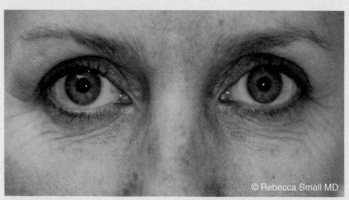

A. Before

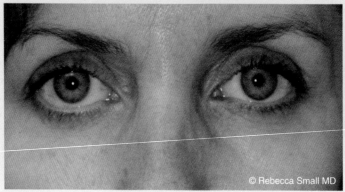

B. After

FIGURE 4-11 ● Infraocular lines before **(A)** and 1 month after **(B)** botulinum toxin treatment using 1.25 units BTX in the inferior palpebral orbicularis oculi m. at rest. (© Rebecca Small MD.)

Follow-ups and Management

Eyelid wrinkles are assessed 2 weeks after botulinum toxin treatment to evaluate for reduction of lower eyelid wrinkles and eyelid position. Persistent lower eyelid wrinkles are often due to one of the following reasons:

- **Deep static wrinkling.** If static wrinkles are present, patients may require several consecutive botulinum toxin treatments for improvements to be seen. Botulinum toxin doses are not routinely escalated in the lower eyelid region because of increased risk of complications with larger doses. Combining botulinum toxin with other minimally invasive aesthetic procedures can enhance results for treatment of static lower eyelid wrinkles (see Combining Aesthetic Treatments and Maximizing Results).
- **Adjacent muscle involvement.** In some patients, lower eyelid wrinkles result from upward movement of the cheek due to contraction of the zygomaticus and/or levator labii superioris muscles. These patients will not benefit from botulinum toxin treatment of the lower eyelid.

Complications and Management

- General injection-related and botulinum toxin-related complications (see Introduction and Foundation Concepts section, Complications)
- Infraocular festoons (eye bags)
- Lower eyelid edema
- Impaired blink reflex
- Ectropion of the lower eyelid (eyelid margin eversion)
- Lagophthalmos (incomplete eyelid closure)
- Xerophthalmia (dry eyes)
- Corneal damage
- Diplopia (double vision)
- Strabismus (crossed eyes)
- Epiphoria (tearing)
- Globe trauma

Infraocular festoons may worsen with botulinum toxin injection in the lower eyelid region due to excessive weakening of the inferior orbicularis oculi muscle.

Lower eyelid edema usually reported as lower eyelid fullness or puffiness, may result from impaired lymphatic drainage due to weakening of the pretarsal orbicularis oculi muscle. Symptoms of lower eyelid edema are typically worse in the morning.

Impaired eyelid function and altered lower eyelid position, such as **ectropion** and **lagophthalmos,** are very rare and can occur with high botulinum toxin doses that excessively weaken the orbicularis oculi m., or if botulinum toxin is placed too close to the eyelid. **Xerophthalmia,** which is extremely rare, can result from impaired eyelid function with reduced lacrimal flow or may be secondary to ectropion and lagophthalmos. Patients who have had LASIK surgery may be more susceptible to xerophthalmia. **Corneal damage** such as keratitis sicca (corneal desiccation) and punctate keratitis (corneal ulcerations) can result from prolonged dry eyes and corneal exposure. **Diplopia** and **strabismus** can occur with deep migration of botulinum toxin into extraocular muscles. **Epiphora** may result from lacrimal dysfunction, if botulinum toxin is placed medial to the midpupillary line. **Globe trauma** is a risk with injections in the lower eyelid area that are usually superior to the bony orbital rim.

There are no corrective treatments for most ocular complications; however, they will spontaneously resolve as botulinum toxin effects diminish. Consultation with an ophthalmologist is advisable with ocular complications.

Botulinum Toxin Treatment of Other Areas

Botulinum toxin treatment of the following areas may further reduce lower eyelid wrinkles:
- **Bunny lines** due to the nasalis m. contraction (see Bunny Lines chapter)
- **Crow's feet** due to lateral orbicularis oculi m. contraction (see Crow's Feet chapter)

Combining Aesthetic Treatments and Maximizing Results

Static lower eyelid wrinkles. Botulinum toxin in the inferiior orbicularuis oculi m. can be combined with the following minimally invasive aesthetic procedures to reduce static lower eyelid wrinkles:
- Resurfacing procedures such as fractional ablative lasers and chemical peels are helpful adjunctive treatments.
- Topical products such as retinoids (eg, tretinoin), growth factors, and alpha hydroxy acids (eg, glycolic and lactic acid) have been shown to reduce fine lines when used consistently over a period of months. Prescription strength retinoids are associated with a retinoid dermatitis, and other less irritative products, such as over the counter retinol, are more commonly used in the periocular area.

Pricing

Charges for botulinum toxin treatment of lower eyelid wrinkles range from $75-$100 per treatment or $50-$60 per unit. This area is typically treated concomitantly with crow's feet.

Case Studies

The techniques in this chapter for botulinum toxin treatment of the inferior orbicularis oculi m. are applied to patients with a variety of presentations encountered in clinical practice in the Cases section.

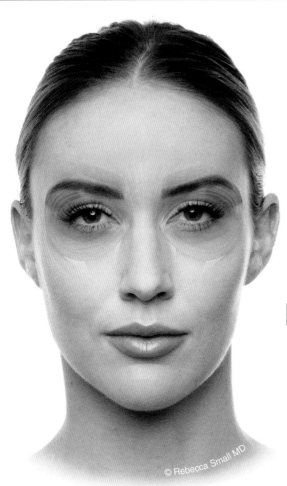

© Rebecca Small MD

Eyebrow Lift

Low-positioned eyebrows (eyebrow ptosis) and eyelid skin laxity (dermatochalasis) convey a fatigued or sad appearance and are accentuated by contraction of the supero-lateral orbicularis oculi muscle. These conditions can often be improved with botulinum toxin treatment of the superolateral orbicularis oculi m., which inhibits muscle contraction and elevates the lateral eyebrow. Elevation of the lateral eyebrow is called an eyebrow lift or chemical brow lift. Treatment of other muscle groups in the upper face can also elevate eyebrows (see Combining Aesthetic Treatments and Maximizing Results at the end of this chapter); however, botulinum toxin treatment of the supero-lateral orbicularis oculi m. is the focus of this chapter.

Anatomy

- **Eyebrow position and shape.** In women, the ideal eyebrow position is slightly above the supraorbital ridge and the eyebrow has an arched, gull-wing shape that tapers (Fig. 5-1A). In men, eyebrows are positioned at the supraorbital ridge and are flat in shape (Fig. 5-1B).
- **Wrinkles.** Infrabrow wrinkles radiate superolaterally from the eye to the eyebrow (see Fig. 3-1, Crow's Feet chapter).

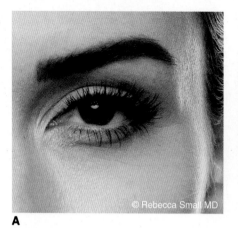
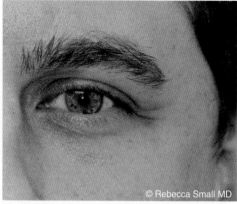

A   **B**

FIGURE 5-1 ● Eyebrow shape in women **(A)** and men **(B)**. (© Rebecca Small MD.)

- **Muscles targeted.** Lateral eyebrow lift and reduction of dermatochalasis and infrabrow wrinkles with botulinum toxin target the superolateral orbital portion of the orbicularis oculi muscle. Other muscles in the upper face affecting eyebrow height and position and are listed in Table 5-1 (see Anatomy section, Figs. 1 to 3 and Lower Eyelid Wrinkles chapter, Fig. 4-2).
- **Muscle functions.** Contraction of the superolateral orbicularis oculi m. lowers the lateral eyebrow, aids in closure of the eyelid and lacrimal function, and forms infrabrow wrinkles (see Anatomy section, Fig. 7).

Patient Assessment

- **General patient assessment** and **consultation** principles are outlined in the Introduction (see Introduction and Foundation Concepts section, Patient Selection and Aesthetic Consultation).
- **Eyebrow ptosis** and **upper eyelid dermatochalasis** or skin laxity (also referred to as "hooding") are assessed with the frontalis m. at rest. Patients with severe dermatochalasis who have excessive folds with lax skin resting on the upper eyelid, or severe eyebrow ptosis, typically do not show significant improvement with a botulinum toxin eyebrow lift alone. These patients may require botulinum toxin treatment of other adjacent muscles (see Botulinum Toxin Treatment of Other Areas), or more aggressive surgical interventions such as blepharoplasty or a forehead lift.

TABLE 5-1

Effects of Muscle Contraction and Botulinum Toxin Treatments on Eyebrow Height and Shape

Muscle	Muscle Effect on Eyebrow	Botulinum Toxin Effect on Eyebrow
Glabellar complex	Medial eyebrow depressor	Elevates medial eyebrow
Superolateral orbicularis oculi	Lateral eyebrow depressor	Elevates lateral eyebrow
Lateral orbicularis oculi	Lateral eyebrow depressor	Elevates lateral eyebrow
Frontalis	Medial and lateral eyebrow levator	Lowers medial and lateral eyebrow

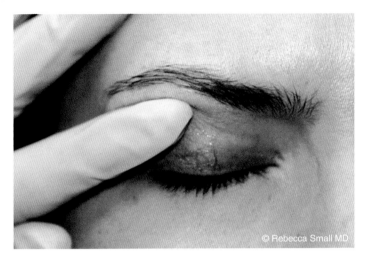

FIGURE 5-2 ● Superolateral orbicularis muscle targeted with botulinum toxin eyebrow lift treatments. (© Rebecca Small MD.)

- **Superolateral orbicularis oculi muscle strength** is assessed by placing the index finger beneath this portion of the muscle and having the patient contract the muscle (Fig. 5-2). If the patient can exert forceful downward pressure against the finger producing a visible roll of contracted muscle, the eyebrow lift procedure will typically yield noticeable elevation of the lateral eyebrow in the absence of severe eyebrow ptosis and severe dermatochalasis.
- **Concomitant muscle contraction in other facial areas** is assessed with superolateral orbicularis oculi m. contraction. Treatment of eyebrow depressors including the glabellar complex (see Frown Lines chapter), lateral orbicularis oculi m. (see Crow's Feet chapter) and in some patients, nasalis m. (see Bunny Lines chapter) concomitantly with the superolateral orbicularis oculi m. is usually necessary to achieve optimal eyebrow height and shape.

 Tip

Discuss opposing levator and depressor actions on the eyebrows at the time of consultation so patients understand the rationale behind treating adjacent muscles to help achieve desired eyebrow height and shape.

Contraindications

- General contraindications to botulinum toxin treatments are listed in the Introduction (see Introduction and Foundation Concepts section, Contraindications).

Eliciting Contraction of the Muscles to Be Treated

Instruct the patient to perform the following expression:
- "Blink hard and hold it"

Treatment Goal

- Partial inhibition of the superolateral orbicularis oculi muscle.

Reconstitution

- Botulinum toxin is abbreviated as BTX in this book and refers to onabotulinumtoxinA (Botox®), incobotulinumtoxinA (Xeomin®), and prabotulinumtoxinA (Jeuveau®). These products have similar 1:1 dosing ratios.
- Reconstitute 100 units of BTX powder with 4 mL of nonpreserved sterile saline (see Introduction and Foundation Concepts section, Reconstitution Method).

Starting Doses

- Women: total (bilateral) dose is 5-7.5 units BTX
- Men: total (bilateral) dose is 7.5-10 units BTX

 Tip

Maximum combined botulinum toxin dose recommended for all treatments in a single session is 100 units BTX for providers just getting started, and may be greater than 100 units BTX per session for experienced providers.

Anesthesia

- Anesthesia is not necessary for most patients but an ice pack may be used if required.

Equipment for Treatment

- General botulinum toxin injection supplies (see Introduction and Foundation Concepts section, Equipment)
- Reconstituted botulinum toxin
- 30-gauge, 0.5-in needle

Procedure Overview

- Place injections in the eyebrow lift Safety Zone (Fig. 5-3). The Safety Zone is bounded by the supraorbital ridge and is at least 1 cm superior to the orbital rim and 1 cm lateral to the lateral iris line.

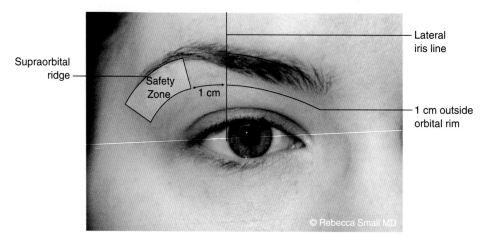

FIGURE 5-3 ● Eyebrow lift Safety Zone for botulinum toxin treatments. (© Rebecca Small MD.)

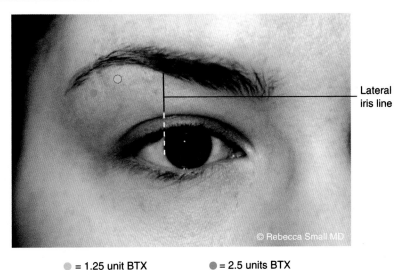

Lateral
iris line

 = 1.25 unit BTX   = 2.5 units BTX

FIGURE 5-4 ● Overview of botulinum toxin injection sites and doses for lateral eyebrow lift. (© Rebecca Small MD.)

- An overview of injection sites and botulinum toxin doses for a lateral eyebrow lift is shown in Figure 5-4.
- Botulinum toxin is injected intramuscularly with the eyebrow lift procedure.

Tip

Injecting superolateral to the Safety Zone can increase the risk of eyebrow ptosis (droopy upper eyebrow) due to botulinum toxin weakening the frontalis muscle.

Tip

Injecting superomedial to the Safety Zone can increase the risk of blepharoptosis (droopy upper eyelid) due to botulinum toxin weakening the levator palpebrae superioris muscle (see Frown Lines chapter).

Technique

1. Position the patient at a 60° angle.
2. Identify the eyebrow lift Safety Zone (Fig. 5-3).
3. Identify the superolateral portion of the orbicularis oculi m. by instructing the patient to contract the muscle as described above and palpate the roll of contracted muscle (Fig. 5-2).
4. Identify the injection sites (Fig. 5-4).
5. Ice for anesthesia (optional).
6. Prepare injection sites with alcohol and allow to dry.
7. The provider is positioned on the side that is to be injected.
8. While the orbicularis oculi m. is relaxed, insert the needle in the first injection site located approximately 1.5 cm lateral to the lateral iris line, within the Safety Zone (Fig. 5-5). Direct the needle superiorly toward the forehead and angle away from the lateral iris line. Using superficial intramuscular placement, inject 2.5 units BTX.

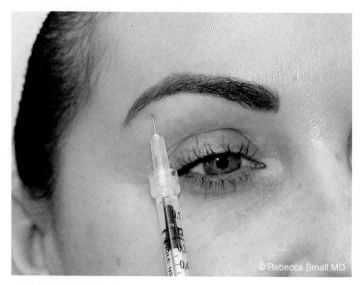

FIGURE 5-5 ● Lateral eyebrow lift botulinum toxin injection technique.
(© Rebecca Small MD.)

9. The second injection site is 1 cm medial to the first injection site, closer to the lateral iris line. Insert the needle similarly and inject 1.25 units BTX.
10. Repeat the above injections for the contralateral side of the face.
11. Compress the injection sites firmly, directing pressure away from the eye.

 Tip

Total number of botulinum toxin injection sites for treatment of the superolateral orbicularis oculi m. to lift the lateral eyebrow is typically 4.

Results

• **Lateral eyebrow elevation** and reduction of **upper eyelid dermatochalasis** is typically seen 3-5 days after botulinum toxin treatment, with maximal improvement at 2 weeks. Figure 5-6 shows a patient at rest before (Fig. 5-6A) and 2 weeks after (Fig. 5-6B) botulinum toxin injection demonstrating eyebrow elevation with reduction of dermatochalasis.

Duration of Effects and Treatment Intervals

• Muscle function in the treatment area gradually returns 2-3 months after botulinum toxin treatment.
• Eyebrow lifting is subtle and determining when to return for treatment can be challenging for patients. Subsequent treatments may be performed when eyebrow descent is noticeable or when patients notice recurrence of eyelid heaviness or a fatigued appearance. The author typically performs an eyebrow lift every 3-4 months with the same time intervals as other upper face botulinum toxin treatments.

RESULTS

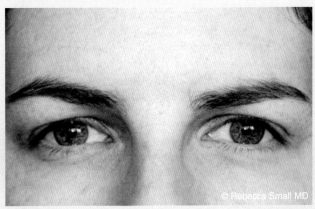

A. Before

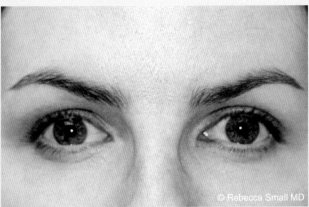

B. After

FIGURE 5-6 ● Eyebrow lift before **(A)** and 2 weeks after **(B)** botulinum toxin treatment using 7.5 units BTX in the superolateral orbicularis oculi m. and 20 units BTX in the glabellar complex muscles, at rest. (© Rebecca Small MD.)

Follow-ups and Management

Eyebrow symmetry, shape, and height are assessed at a 2-week visit after botulinum toxin treatment.
- **Additional lateral eyebrow elevation.** If additional lateral eyebrow elevation is desired, assess the strength of the superolateral orbicularis oculi muscle. If significant contractility is still present, additional botulinum toxin may be injected in the same areas previously treated. Total bilateral dose for this touch-up procedure is usually 2.5-5 units BTX.

Complications and Management

- General injection-related and botulinum toxin-related complications (see Introduction and Foundation Concepts section, Complications)
- Blepharoptosis (droopy eye lid)
- Lack of eyebrow elevation

Blepharoptosis may occur as a complication from eyebrow lift treatments, particularly if botulinum toxin is injected too close to the supraorbital ridge at the lateral iris line. Blepharoptosis results from migration of botulinum toxin through the orbital septum fascia to the levator palpebrae superioris m. in the upper eyelid. Some of the levator palpebrae superioris m. fibers pass up through the orbital septum to attach on the supraorbital ridge at the lateral iris. Botulinum toxin can migrate into the levator palpebrae superioris m. at this "weak point." See Frown Lines chapter, Complications and Management, for additional information on blepharoptosis and management strategies. Angling the needle away from the lateral iris line with injections can reduce the risk of blepharoptosis from botulinum toxin treatment of the superolateral orbicularis oculi muscle.

Lack of eyebrow elevation may occur if other eyebrow depressors (ie, glabellar complex, lateral orbicularis oculi, and in some patients nasalis muscles) are not treated along with the superolateral orbicularis oculi muscle. These other muscles are comparatively larger and stronger, and treating them with botulinum toxin to balance the levator-depressor effects on the eyebrow is usually necessary to achieve optimal eyebrow height and shape.

 Tip

Blepharoptosis can result from botulinum toxin diffusion to the levator palabrae superioris m. that elevates the upper eyelid in two main ways: (1) superior injection in the glabellar complex when treating frown lines, and (2) inferior injection in the superolateral orbicularis oculi m. when performing an eyebrow lift.

Botulinum Toxin Treatment of Other Areas

Combining botulinum toxin treatments in multiple muscles of the upper face optimizes eyebrow shape and height and enhances lifting of different portions of the eyebrow as follows:
- **Glabellar complex** (see Frown Lines chapter) for additional medial eyebrow elevation
- **Lateral orbicularis oculi muscle** (see Crow's Feet chapter) for additional lateral eyebrow elevation
- **Frontalis muscle**, using the "V-shaped" injection pattern (see Horizontal Forehead Lines chapter) for additional lateral eyebrow elevation

Combining Aesthetic Treatments and Maximizing Results

Additional eyebrow lifting. Lateral eyebrow elevation can also be enhanced by combining botulinum toxin lateral eyebrow lift with infrabrow dermal filler treatment (see *A Practical Guide to Dermal Filler Procedures*).

Pricing

Charges for botulinum toxin eyebrow lift treatments range from $150-$200 per treatment or $10-$25 per unit of BTX.

Case Studies

The techniques in this chapter for botulinum toxin treatment of the superolateral orbicularis oculi m. are applied to patients with a variety of presentations encountered in clinical practice in the Cases section.

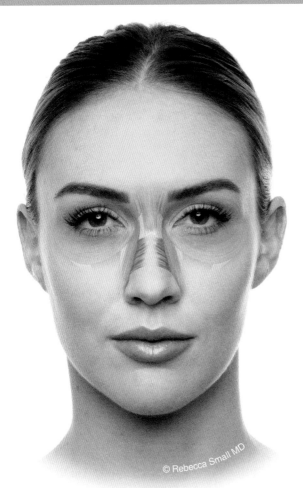

Chapter 6

© Rebecca Small MD

Bunny Lines

Dynamic bunny lines result from contraction of the nasalis muscle. While some patients associate these lines with distaste and disapproval, others are unconcerned with bunny lines. Botulinum toxin treatment of the nasalis m. reduces bunny lines, including horizontal lines at the root of the nose, by inhibiting muscle contraction and smoothing the overlying skin.

Anatomy

- **Wrinkles.** Bunny lines, or nasalis rhytids, are wrinkles on the lateral and dorsal aspects of the nose formed by frowning, smiling, and squinting. They typically course diagonally over the nasal sidewalls and vertically over the mid to lower nasal bridge (Fig. 6-6A and see Anatomy section, Figs. 4, 5, and 8).
- **Muscles targeted.** Botulinum toxin bunny line treatment targets the nasalis muscle (see Anatomy section, Figs. 1 to 3). Nasalis m. fibers can interdigitate with the procerus and the medial orbicularis oculi muscles.
- **Muscle functions.** Nasalis contraction draws the nasal sidewalls superiorly and medially, producing bunny lines (see Anatomy section, Fig. 7). In some cases nasalis m. contraction contributes to formation of horizontal lines at the root of the nose (Fig. 6-1)

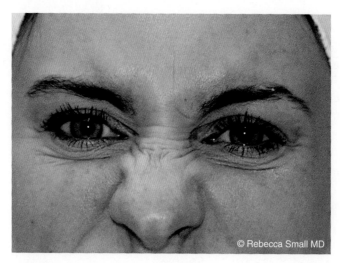

FIGURE 6-1 ● Transverse nasal lines due to contraction of the procerus muscle. (© Rebecca Small MD.)

due to concomitant contraction with the procerus m. when frowning, and medial lower eyelid wrinkles due to contraction of the orbicularis oculi m. when smiling.

- **Muscles avoided.** The levator labii superioris alaeque nasi m. (LLSAN) that lies on the lateral border of the nasalis m. can also contribute to formation of bunny lines. This is primarily an upper lip levator and is avoided with treatment of bunny lines (see Anatomy section, Figs. 1 to 3).

Patient Assessment

- **General patient assessment** and **consultation** principles are outlined in the Introduction (see Introduction and Foundation Concepts section, Patient Selection and Aesthetic Consultation).
- **Dynamic** (with muscle contraction) and **static** (at rest) **bunny lines** are assessed.
- **Concomitant muscle contraction in other facial areas** is assessed. Patients that form bunny lines when frowning (see Frown Lines chapter) or smiling (see Crow's Feet chapter) can experience compensatory contraction the nasalis m. with worsening bunny lines if the nasalis m. is not treated concomitantly with these other muscles. Horizontal lines at the root of the nose usually require concomitant treatment of the nasalis and glabellar complex muscles.

Contraindications

- General contraindications to botulinum toxin treatments are listed in the Introduction (see Introduction and Foundation Concepts section, Contraindications).

Eliciting Contraction of Muscles to Be Treated

Instruct the patient to perform the following expression:
- "Think of a bad skunk smell"
- "Scrunch your nose"

Treatment Goal

- Complete inhibition of the nasalis muscle.

Reconstitution

- Botulinum toxin is abbreviated as BTX in this book and refers to onabotulinumtoxinA (Botox®), incobotulinumtoxinA (Xeomin®), and prabotulinumtoxinA (Jeuveau®). These products have similar 1:1 dosing ratios.
- Reconstitute 100 units BTX powder with 4 mL of nonpreserved sterile saline (see Introduction and Foundation Concepts section, Reconstitution Method).

Starting Doses

- Women and men: 3.75-5 units BTX

 Tip

Maximum combined botulinum toxin dose recommended for all treatments in a single session is 100 units BTX for providers just getting started, and may be greater than 100 units BTX per session for experienced providers.

Anesthesia

- Application of a topical anesthetic such as BLT (see Introduction and Foundation Concepts section, Anesthesia) and an ice pack is helpful to reduce discomfort in this sensitive area.

Equipment for Treatment

- General botulinum toxin injection supplies (see Introduction and Foundation Concepts section, Equipment)
- Reconstituted botulinum toxin
- 30-gauge, 0.5-in needle

Procedure Overview

- Place injections within the bunny line Safety Zone (Fig. 6-2A and B). The Safety Zone is a region bounded superiorly by the nasion (the least protruding part of the nose between the medial canthi); and inferiorly at a point located halfway between the nasion and nasal tip. It is bounded laterally by the nasion-ala line, which extends from the edge of the nasal ala along the nasal side wall, up to the nasion line. In general, the inferior Safety Zone point lies at the inferior most bunny line.
- An overview of injection sites and botulinum toxin doses for treatment of bunny lines is shown in Figure 6-3.
- Botulinum toxin is injected subdermally for treatment of bunny lines.

 Tip

Injecting lateral to the Safety Zone can increase the risk of upper lip ptosis (droopy upper lip) due to botulinum toxin weakening the levator labii superioris alaeque nasi muscle (LLSAN).

Technique

1. Position the patient at a 60° angle.
2. Identify the bunny line Safety Zone (Fig. 6-2).
3. Locate the nasalis m. by instructing the patient to contract the muscles using one of the facial expressions above.
4. Identify the injection sites (Fig. 6-3).
5. Apply topical anesthetic and ice for anesthesia as needed.
6. Prepare injection sites with alcohol and allow to dry.
7. The provider is positioned on the side that is to be injected.
8. While the nasalis m. is contracted, insert the needle medial to the nasion-ala line on the nasal sidewall within the Safety Zone (Fig. 6-4). Angle the needle toward the nasal sidewall and insert subdermally. Inject 1.25 units BTX.
9. Repeat the above injection on the contralateral nasal wall.

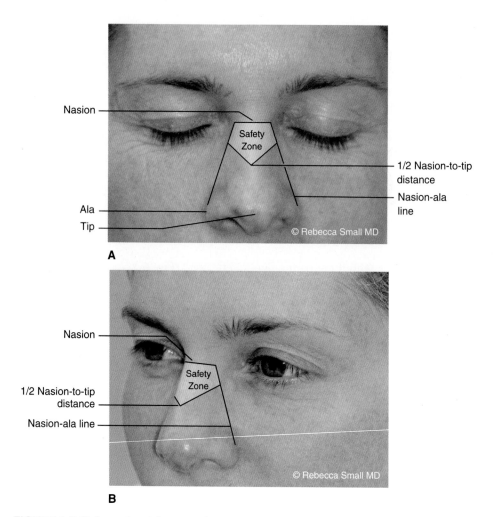

FIGURE 6-2 ● Bunny line Safety Zone for botulinum toxin treatments: anterior-posterior **(A)** and oblique **(B)** views. (© Rebecca Small MD.)

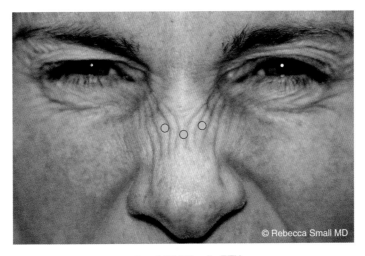

 = 1.25-2.5 units BTX

FIGURE 6-3 ● Overview of botulinum toxin injection sites and doses for treatment of bunny lines. (© Rebecca Small MD.)

10. The third injection site is on the dorsum of the nose. Reposition to stand in front of the patient. With the nasalis m. contracted, approach inferiorly, angling the needle toward the dorsum of the nose, and inject 1.25 units BTX (Fig. 6-5).
11. Compress injection wheals medially.

👆 Tip

Total number of botulinum toxin injection sites for treatment of the nasalis m. to reduce bunny lines is typically 3-4.

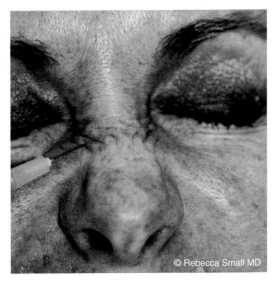

FIGURE 6-4 ● Nasalis m. sidewall botulinum toxin injection technique. (© Rebecca Small MD.)

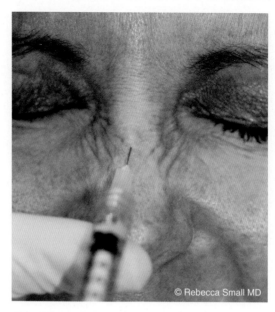

FIGURE 6-5 ● Nasalis m. dorsum botulinum toxin injection technique. (© Rebecca Small MD.)

Results

- **Reduction of dynamic bunny lines** is typically seen 3-5 days after botulinum toxin treatment, with maximal improvement at 2 weeks. Figure 6-6 shows contraction of the nasalis m. before (Fig. 6-6A) and 2 weeks after (Fig. 6-6B) botulinum toxin injection.

Duration of Effects and Treatment Intervals

- Muscle function in the treatment area gradually returns 3-4 months after botulinum toxin treatment.
- Subsequent bunny line treatments with botulinum toxin may be performed when the nasalis m. begins to contract, before the lines return to their pretreatment appearance.

Follow-ups and Management

Bunny lines are assessed 2-weeks after botulinum toxin treatment to evaluate for reduced bunny lines. If persistent bunny lines are present, evaluate for one of the following common causes:

- **Persistent nasalis muscle contraction.** Some patients may have greater muscle mass than anticipated in the treatment area and additional botulinum toxin may be required to achieve desired results. Persistent muscle contraction can be corrected with a touch-up procedure using 1.25-2.5 units BTX, depending on the degree of nasalis m. activity present.
- **Static lines.** If static lines are present, patients may require several consecutive botulinum toxin treatments for results to be seen.

RESULTS

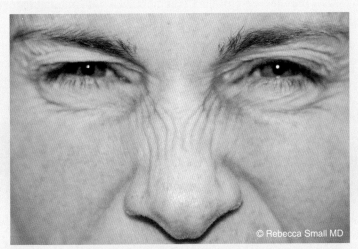

A. Before

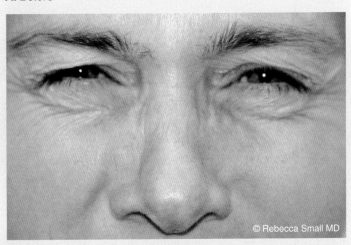

B. After

FIGURE 6-6 ● Bunny lines before **(A)** and 2 weeks after **(B)** botulinum toxin treatment using 3.75 units BTX in the nasalis m., during maximal contraction. (© Rebecca Small MD.)

Complications and Management

- General injection-related and botulinum toxin-related complications (see Introduction and Foundation Concepts section, Complications)
- Lip ptosis with resultant smile asymmetry
- Oral incompetence with resultant drooling and impaired speaking, eating, or drinking
- Epiphora (excess tearing)
- Diplopia

Lip ptosis and **smile asymmetry** can occur if botulinum toxin affects the adjacent lip levator muscles, particularly the levator labii superioris alaeque nasi muscle (LLSAN). Injections placed too inferiorly, along the nasal sidewall, can involve the levator labii superioris alaeque nasi muscle (LLSAN). Rarely, functional impairments such as **oral incompetence** with drooling, impaired speech, and difficulty eating or drinking may occur if lip levator muscles are profoundly immobilized with botulinum toxin.

Epiphora can result from impaired lacrimal function if the medial palpebral portion of the orbicularis oculi m. is affected. Injections too close to the medial canthus can result in botulinum toxin diffusion to extraocular muscles (eg, medial rectus m.) resulting in **diplopia.** Consultation with an ophthalmologist is advisable for ocular complications.

There are no corrective treatments of these complications; however, they spontaneously resolve as botulinum toxin effects diminish.

Botulinum Toxin Treatment of Other Areas

Bunny lines can be accentuated with botulinum toxin treatment of the **glabellar complex** (see Frown Lines chapter) and **orbicularis oculi m.** (see Crow's Feet chapter). Patients who form bunny lines when engaging these other areas benefit from concomitant botulinum toxin treatment of the nasalis m. to prevent worsening of bunny lines over time.

Combining Aesthetic Treatments and Maximizing Results

Bunny lines typically respond well to botulinum toxin treatments and rarely require combination therapy.

Pricing

Charges for botulinum toxin treatment of bunny lines range from $150-$200 per treatment or $10-$25 per unit of BTX.

Case Studies

The techniques in this chapter for botulinum toxin treatment of the nasalis m. are applied to patients with a variety of presentations encountered in clinical practice in the Cases section.

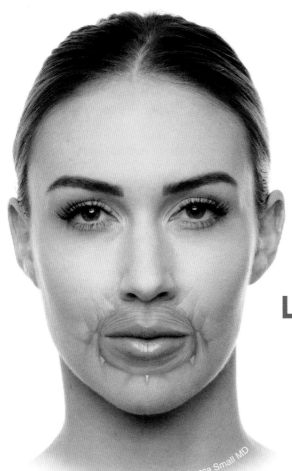

Chapter 7

Key Points

Advanced Treatment Area

Indications: Radial lip lines, Enhanced lip fullness or "lip flip"

Muscles Targeted: Orbicularis oris muscle

Contraindications: Occupations requiring full perioral strength

Lip Lines and Lip Flip

Dynamic lip lines result from contraction of the orbicularis oris muscle. These lines are seen almost exclusively in women and are associated with an aged appearance. Botulinum toxin treatment of the orbicularis oris m. reduces lip lines by inhibiting muscle contraction and smoothing the overlying skin, and enhances lip fullness by everting the upper lip, referred to as a "lip flip." Upper lip lines are a common complaint and, while Safety Zones and injection sites for both upper and lower lips are discussed, the focus of this chapter is botulinum toxin treatment of the upper lip.

Anatomy

- **Wrinkles.** Lip lines, or perioral rhytids, commonly referred to as lipstick lines or smoker's lines are wrinkles that extend radially from the upper and lower lip borders (Figs. 7-4A, 7-6A, 7-7A and see Anatomy section, Figs. 4, 5, and 8).
- **Muscles targeted.** Botulinum toxin lip line treatment targets the orbicularis oris m., a sphincteric muscle that encircles the mouth (see Anatomy section, Figs. 1 to 3).
- **Muscle functions.** The orbicularis oris m. functions to close the lips and to invert the lip border (see Anatomy section, Fig. 7). The orbicularis oris m. contributes to facial expressions such as puckering, and essential functions of speaking, eating, and drinking.

- **Muscles avoided.** Many muscles of the middle and lower face insert and exert effects on the lips and most of these muscles lie deep to the orbicularis oris muscle. Upper lip levator muscles avoided with botulinum toxin treatment of lip lines include levator labii superioris alaeque nasi, levator labii superioris, zygomaticus minor, zygomaticus major, and levator anguli oris (see Anatomy section, Fig. 3).

 Tip

The lower face has numerous small muscles that interdigitate and a detailed understanding of facial anatomy with precise placement of small botulinum toxin doses is required for treatments.

Patient Assessment

- **General patient assessment** and **consultation** principles are outlined in the Introduction (see Introduction and Foundation Concepts section, Patient Selection and Aesthetic Consultation).
- **Social history** is obtained including occupations and activities that require full oral competence, such as wind instrument musicians, actors, singers, and public speakers.
- **Dynamic** (with muscle contraction) and **static** (at rest) **lip lines** are assessed.

Contraindications

- General contraindications to botulinum toxin treatments are listed in the Introduction (see Introduction and Foundation Concepts section, Contraindications).
- Specific contraindications to botulinum toxin treatment of lip lines and lip flip include occupations requiring full perioral strength such as musicians, actors, singers, and public speakers.

Eliciting Contraction of Muscles to Be Treated

Instruct the patient to perform any of the following expressions:
- "Whistle"
- "Sip on a straw"
- "Pucker"

Treatment Goal

- Partial inhibition of the upper lip orbicularis oris m. to reduce lip lines with avoidance of the philtral area to maintain a desirable lip shape and preservation of essential perioral function.

 Tip

Adequate strength must be maintained in the orbicularis oris m. with botulinum toxin treatments so that essential functions of speaking, eating, and drinking are preserved.

Reconstitution

- Botulinum toxin is abbreviated as BTX in this book and refers to onabotulinumtoxinA (Botox®), incobotulinumtoxinA (Xeomin®), and prabotulinumtoxinA (Jeuveau®). These products have similar 1:1 dosing ratios.
- Reconstitute 100 units of BTX powder with 4 mL of nonpreserved sterile saline (see Introduction and Foundation Concepts section, Reconstitution Method).

Starting Doses

- Women and men: total (bilateral) dose is 3.75-5 units BTX for the upper lip

> ✋ **Tip**
>
> Maximum combined botulinum toxin dose recommended for all treatments in a single session is 100 units BTX for providers just getting started, and may be greater than 100 units BTX per session for experienced providers.

Anesthesia

- The upper lip is very sensitive and anesthesia is required. Topical anesthetic reduces motor function in the applied area and, therefore, is applied after evaluating the area for dynamic wrinkling and taking photographs.
- Apply a topical anesthetic such as benzocaine/lidocaine/tetracaine (BLT) without occlusion for 15 minutes before treatment (see Introduction and Foundation Concepts section, Anesthesia).
- In addition, application of ice for 1-2 minutes immediately before treatment is also recommended.

Equipment for Treatment

- General botulinum toxin injection supplies (see Introduction and Foundation Concepts section, Equipment)
- Reconstituted botulinum toxin
- 30-gauge, 0.5-in needle

Procedure Overview

- Place injections in the lip line Safety Zone (Fig. 7-1).
  - **Upper lip line Safety Zone** is at least 1 cm from the lateral corners of the mouth, 0.5 cm or less from the vermillion border, and extends to the lateral edge of the philtral column (Fig. 7-1A).
  - **Lower lip line Safety Zone** is at least 2 cm from the lateral corners of the mouth and is 0.5 cm or less from the vermillion border (Fig. 7-1B).
- An overview of injection sites and botulinum toxin doses for treatment of lip lines is shown in Figure 7-2. The upper lip requires one injection per side (Fig. 7-2A). The lower lip typically requires one injection across the midline (Fig. 7-2B).
- Marking injection sites with the muscle contracted before anesthesia is helpful because once anesthetized, patients are unable to contract this muscle.
- Botulinum toxin is injected subdermally using a threading technique for treatment.
- In patients who have never had botulinum toxin treatment of the lips, and for providers who are getting started with lip line botulinum toxin treatments, it is advisable to treat only the upper or the lower lip in a given visit.

> ✋ **Tip**
>
> Injecting lateral to the lip line Safety Zone or too deep may increase the risk of oral incompetence due to botulinum toxin weakening the muscles that control lip function.

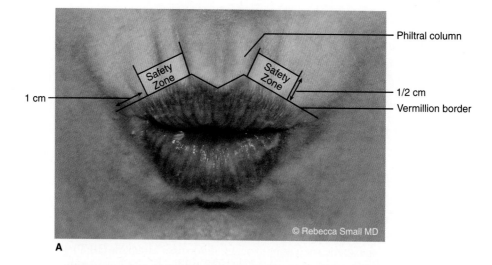

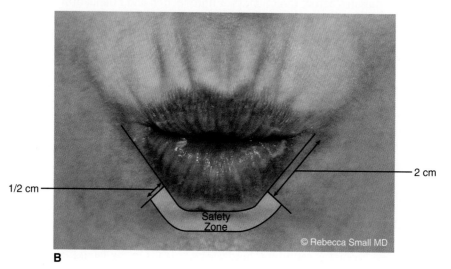

FIGURE 7-1 ● Lip line Safety Zones for the upper lip **(A)** and lower lip **(B)**, with botulinum toxin treatments. (© Rebecca Small MD.)

 Tip

Injecting medial to the lip line Safety Zone, into the philtral columns, may result in an undesired flattening of the Cupid's bow.

Technique

1. Position the patient at a 60° angle.
2. Identify the lip line Safety Zone (Fig. 7-1).
3. Locate the orbicularis oris m. by instructing the patient to contract the muscle using one of the facial expressions above.
4. Identify the injection sites (Fig. 7-2). With the orbicularis oris m. contracted, mark the two injection sites on the upper lip in the ridges of the muscle, near the vermillion border, at least 1 cm away from the corners of the mouth.
5. Apply topical anesthetic to the treatment area for 10-15 minutes and remove before injection.

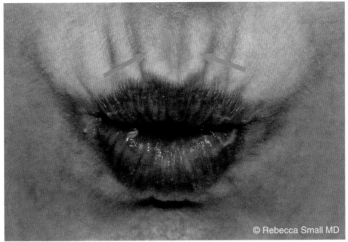

A   ↑ = 2.5 units BTX, insert needle in direction of arrow

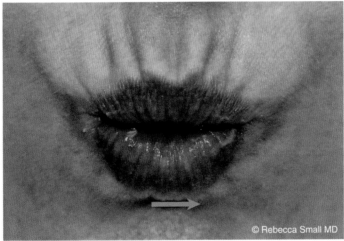

B   ↑ = 2.5 units BTX, insert needle in direction of arrow

FIGURE 7-2 ● Overview of botulinum toxin injection sites and doses in the upper **(A)** and lower **(B)** lips for treatment of lip lines and enhanced lip fullness. (© Rebecca Small MD.)

6. Apply ice for anesthesia immediately prior to injection on the side of the upper lip to be treated.
7. Prepare injection sites with alcohol and allow to dry.
8. The provider is positioned on the side that is to be injected.
9. While the mouth is at rest, insert the needle into the first injection site and thread superficially, such that the needle tip ends 1-2 mm lateral to the edge of the philtral column. Use the first finger of the noninjecting hand to gently palpate the needle tip in the tissue and confirm placement. Inject 2.5 units with gentle, even plunger pressure as the needle is withdrawn (Fig. 7-3).
10. Compress the injection sites firmly to relieve discomfort.
11. Apply ice for anesthesia to the contralateral side of the upper lip to be treated.
12. Prepare injection sites with alcohol and allow to dry.
13. Repeat the above technique for the contralateral side of the upper lip.

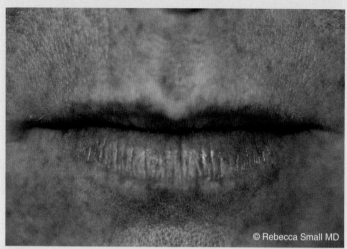

A. Before

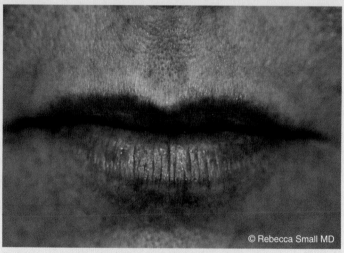

B. After

FIGURE 7-5 ● "Lip flip" before **(A)** and 2 weeks after **(B)** botulinum toxin treatment of the upper orbicularis oris m. at rest. (© Rebecca Small MD.)

that demonstrate dynamic muscle ridges. Reassess patients 2 weeks after the touch-up. The efficacious dose of botulinum toxin for treatment of the upper lip is determined to be the initial dose plus the touch-up dose. Start with this total dose at the patient's subsequent upper lip treatment in approximately 2-3 months.

- **Static lines**. If static lines are present, patients may require several consecutive botulinum toxin treatments for improvements to be seen. Combining botulinum toxin with other minimally invasive aesthetic procedures can offer enhanced results for treatment of static lip lines (see Combining Aesthetic Treatments and Maximizing Results).